Sports Injuries

Recent Titles in
Q&A Health Guides

Sports Injuries

❖❖

Your Questions Answered

James H. Johnson

Q&A Health Guides

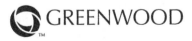

GREENWOOD

An Imprint of ABC-CLIO, LLC
Santa Barbara, California • Denver, Colorado

Library of Congress Cataloging-in-Publication Data

Names: Johnson, James H., author.
Title: Sports injuries : your questions answered / James H. Johnson.
Description: Santa Barbara, California : Greenwood, [2021] | Series: Q&A
   health guides | Includes bibliographical references and index.
Identifiers: LCCN 2021008324 (print) | LCCN 2021008325 (ebook) | ISBN
   9781440875632 (hardcover) | ISBN 9781440875649 (ebook)
Subjects: LCSH: Sports injuries. | Sports injuries—Miscellanea.
Classification: LCC RD97 .J64 2021 (print) | LCC RD97 (ebook) | DDC
   617.1/027—dc23
LC record available at https://lccn.loc.gov/2021008324
LC ebook record available at https://lccn.loc.gov/2021008325

ISBN: 978-1-4408-7563-2 (print)
        978-1-4408-7564-9 (ebook)

25 24 23 22 21   1 2 3 4 5

This book is also available as an eBook.

Greenwood
An Imprint of ABC-CLIO, LLC

ABC-CLIO, LLC
147 Castilian Drive
Santa Barbara, California 93117
www.abc-clio.com

This book is printed on acid-free paper ∞

Manufactured in the United States of America

To my team—Carolyn, Cheryl, Scott, Luke, Zoe, Emmett, Oliver

Contents

Series Foreword

All of us have questions about our health. Is this normal? Should I be doing something differently? Whom should I talk to about my concerns? And our modern world is full of answers. Thanks to the Internet, there's a wealth of information at our fingertips, from forums where people can share their personal experiences to Wikipedia articles to the full text of medical studies. But finding the right information can be an intimidating and difficult task—some sources are written at too high a level, others have been oversimplified, while still others are heavily biased or simply inaccurate.

Q&A Health Guides address the needs of readers who want accurate, concise answers to their health questions, authored by reputable and objective experts, and written in clear and easy-to-understand language. This series focuses on the topics that matter most to young adult readers, including various aspects of physical and emotional well-being as well as other components of a healthy lifestyle. These guides will also serve as a valuable tool for parents, school counselors, and others who may need to answer teens' health questions.

All books in the series follow the same format to make finding information quick and easy. Each volume begins with an essay on health literacy and why it is so important when it comes to gathering and evaluating health information. Next, the top five myths and misconceptions that surround the topic are dispelled. The heart of each guide is a collection of questions and answers, organized thematically. A selection of five case studies provides real-world examples to illuminate key concepts. Rounding out each volume are a directory of resources, glossary, and index.

It is our hope that the books in this series will not only provide valuable information but will also help guide readers toward a lifetime of healthy decision making.

Acknowledgments

The author wishes to thank Maxine Taylor for her expert editing and advice. The author also wishes to thank Carolyn Johnson and Luke Johnson for multiple readings and advice on content.

Introduction

Regular participation in exercise and sport has tremendous benefit not only to our health but also to our quality of life. Sport provides the play and socialization that people need. Regular exercise helps us tune in to our physicality, to appreciate our bodies, to challenge us, to maintain our physical selves. A deterrent to these numerous benefits is a sport injury. Sport injuries can range from mild discomfort to a serious incident that has lifelong consequences. One of the most common reasons for stopping an exercise program is injury. Yet with the possibility of these drawbacks, the benefits of exercise far outweigh the risk.

One of the best strategies to avoid injury is education, to understand how injury might occur and to avoid behaviors that lead to injury. There are clear-cut strategies for reducing the incidence of injury. Regardless of any prevention approach one might use, injuries occur. When this happens, how you deal with the injury affects the outcome. Understanding the etiology of the injury, the cause, helps one prevent future problems.

One solution to the best care and reduction of injury is fact-based research. In this book, information from applied sports medicine research is assimilated and presented in a readable format. All too often in sports medicine, anecdotal information is shared as if it is the truth. Unfortunately, many people involved in leadership positions do not have the training to provide the facts. There is a plethora of coaches and personal trainers throughout the country who provide sports medicine information to athletes and clients. Many times, these individuals have solid educational backgrounds to support their advice. Personal trainers certified by the American College of Sports Medicine or the National Strength and Conditioning Association undergo an arduous certification process, but attending a weekend workshop certifies some personal trainers. In addition, there is no overarching requirement for coaches in the United States. Some coaches are highly trained, while others may act as coaches simply because they were athletes.

This book is not written for professional athletes but for the general public who exercise and play sports. The approach is moderate, doable, and healthy. The central message relates to how to take care of oneself and how to practice healthy sport and exercise. "More is not better" is one of the central themes of the book. Exercise is a good thing, but too much just results in injury. Exercise is not a cure-all; it is just one of several health behaviors that results in improved health and wellness. Overdoing exercise does not result in increased health.

There is no one sport or exercise that is best for everyone. The secret is to find that exercise that you will do, that won't hurt you, and that you enjoy. Exercise and sport should result in joy not pain. You should finish an exercise session feeling good, a sense of accomplishment, and ready to come back. A moderate educated approach to exercise and sport is the key to achieving this.

Guide to Health Literacy

On her 13th birthday, Samantha was diagnosed with type 2 diabetes. She consulted her mom and her aunt, both of whom also have type 2 diabetes, and decided to go with their strategy of managing diabetes by taking insulin. As a result of participating in an after-school program at her middle school that focused on health literacy, she learned that she can help manage the level of glucose in her bloodstream by counting her carbohydrate intake, following a diabetic diet, and exercising regularly. But, what exactly should she do? How does she keep track of her carbohydrate intake? What is a diabetic diet? How long should she exercise and what type of exercise should she do? Samantha is a visual learner, so she turned to her favorite source of media, YouTube, to answer these questions. She found videos from individuals around the world sharing their experiences and tips, doctors (or at least people who have "Dr." in their YouTube channel names), government agencies such as the National Institutes of Health, and even video clips from cat lovers who have cats with diabetes. With guidance from the librarian and the health and science teachers at her school, she assessed the credibility of the information in these videos and even compared their suggestions to some of the print resources that she was able to find at her school library. Now, she knows exactly how to count her carbohydrate level, how to prepare and follow a diabetic diet, and how much (and what) exercise is needed daily. She intends to share her findings with her mom and her aunt, and now she wants to create a chart that summarizes what she has learned that she can share with her doctor.

Samantha's experience is not unique. She represents a shift in our society; an individual no longer views himself or herself as a passive recipient of medical care but as an active mediator of his or her own health. However, in this era when any individual can post his or her opinions and experiences with a particular health condition online with just a few clicks or publish a memoir, it is vital that people know how to assess the credibility of health information. Gone are the days when "publishing" health information required intense vetting. The health information landscape is highly saturated, and people have innumerable sources where they can find information about practically any health topic. The sources (whether print, online, or a person) that an individual consults for health information are crucial because the accuracy and trustworthiness of the information can potentially affect his or her overall health. The ability to find, select, assess, and use health information constitutes a type of literacy—health literacy—that everyone must possess.

THE DEFINITION AND PHASES OF HEALTH LITERACY

One of the most popular definitions for health literacy comes from Ratzan and Parker (2000), who describe health literacy as "the degree to which individuals have the capacity to obtain, process, and understand basic health information and services needed to make appropriate health decisions." Recent research has extrapolated health literacy into health literacy bits, further shedding light on the multiple phases and literacy practices that are embedded within the multifaceted concept of health literacy. Although this research has focused primarily on online health information seeking, these health literacy bits are needed to successfully navigate both print and online sources. There are six phases of health information seeking: (1) Information Need Identification and Question Formulation, (2) Information Search, (3) Information Comprehension, (4) Information Assessment, (5) Information Management, and (6) Information Use.

The first phase is the *information need identification and question formulation phase*. In this phase, one needs to be able to develop and refine a range of questions to frame one's search and understand relevant health terms. In the second phase, *information search*, one has to possess appropriate searching skills, such as using proper keywords and correct spelling in search terms, especially when using search engines and databases. It is also crucial to understand how search engines work (i.e., how search results are derived, what the order of the search results means, how to use the snippets that are provided in the search results list to select websites, and how to determine which listings are ads on a search engine results page). One also has to limit reliance on surface characteristics, such as the design of a website or a book (a website or book that appears to have a lot of information or looks aesthetically pleasant does not necessarily mean it has good information) and language used (a website or book that utilizes jargon, the keywords that one used to conduct the search, or the word "information" does not necessarily indicate it will have good information). The next phase is *information comprehension*, whereby one needs to have the ability to read, comprehend, and recall the information (including textual, numerical, and visual content) one has located from the books and/or online resources.

To assess the credibility of health information (*information assessment* phase), one needs to be able to evaluate information for accuracy, evaluate how current the information is (e.g., when a website was last updated or when a book was published), and evaluate the creators of the source—for example, examine site sponsors or type of sites (.com, .gov, .edu, or .org) or the author of a book (practicing doctor, a celebrity doctor, a patient of a specific disease, etc.) to determine the believability of the person/ organization providing the information. Such credibility perceptions tend to become generalized, so they must be frequently reexamined (e.g., the belief that a specific news agency always has credible health information needs continuous vetting). One also needs to evaluate the credibility of the medium (e.g., television, Internet, radio, social media, and book) and evaluate—not just accept without questioning—others' claims regarding the validity of a site, book, or other specific source of information. At this stage, one has to "make sense of information gathered from diverse sources by identifying misconceptions, main and supporting ideas, conflicting information, point of view, and biases" (American Association of School Librarians [AASL], 2009, p. 13) and conclude which sources/ information are valid and accurate by using conscious strategies rather than simply using intuitive judgments or "rules of thumb." This phase is the most challenging segment of health information seeking and serves as a determinant of success (or lack thereof) in the information-seeking process. The following section on Sources of Health Information further explains this phase.

The fifth phase is *information management*, whereby one has to organize information that has been gathered in some manner to ensure easy retrieval and use in the future. The last phase is *information use*, in which one will synthesize information found across various resources, draw conclusions, and locate the answer to his or her original question and/ or the content that fulfills the information need. This phase also often involves implementation, such as using the information to solve a health problem; make health-related decisions; identify and engage in behaviors that will help a person to avoid health risks; share the health information found with family members and friends who may benefit from it; and advocate more broadly for personal, family, or community health.

THE IMPORTANCE OF HEALTH LITERACY

The conception of health has moved from a passive view (someone is either well or ill) to one that is more active and process based (someone is working toward preventing or managing disease). Hence, the dominant focus has shifted from doctors and treatments to patients and prevention, resulting in the need to strengthen our ability and confidence (as patients and consumers of health care) to look for, assess, understand, manage, share, adapt, and use health-related information. An individual's health literacy level has been found to predict his or her health status better than age, race, educational attainment, employment status, and income level (National Network of Libraries of Medicine, 2013). Greater health literacy also enables individuals to better communicate with health-care providers such as doctors, nutritionists, and therapists, as they can pose more relevant, informed, and useful questions to health-care providers. Another added advantage of greater health literacy is better information-seeking skills, not only for health but also in other domains, such as completing assignments for school.

SOURCES OF HEALTH INFORMATION: THE GOOD, THE BAD, AND THE IN-BETWEEN

For generations, doctors, nurses, nutritionists, health coaches, and other health professionals have been the trusted sources of health information. Additionally, researchers have found that young adults, when they have health-related questions, typically turn to a family member who has had firsthand experience with a health condition because of their family member's close proximity and because of their past experience with, and trust in, this individual. Expertise should be a core consideration when consulting a person, website, or book for health information. The credentials and background of the person or author and conflicting interests of the author (and his or her organization) must be checked and validated to ensure the likely credibility of the health information they are conveying. While books often have implied credibility because of the peer-review process involved, self-publishing has challenged this credibility, so qualifications of book authors should also be verified. When it comes to health information, currency of the source must also be examined. When examining health information/studies presented, pay attention to the exhaustiveness of research methods utilized to offer recommendations or conclusions. Small and nondiverse sample size is often—but not always—an indication of reduced credibility. Studies that confuse correlation with causation is another potential issue to watch for. Information seekers must also pay attention to the sponsors of the research studies. For example, if a study is sponsored by manufacturers of drug Y and the study recommends that drug Y is the best treatment to manage or cure a disease, this may indicate a lack of objectivity on the part of the researchers.

The Internet is rapidly becoming one of the main sources of health information. Online forums, news agencies, personal blogs, social media sites, pharmacy sites, and celebrity "doctors" are all offering medical and health information targeted to various types of people in regard to all types of diseases and symptoms. There are professional journalists, citizen journalists, hoaxers, and people paid to write fake health news on various sites that may appear to have a legitimate domain name and may even have authors who claim to have professional credentials, such as an MD. All these sites *may* offer useful information or information that appears to be useful and relevant; however, much of the information may be debatable and may fall into gray areas that require readers to discern credibility, reliability, and biases.

While broad recognition and acceptance of certain media, institutions, and people often serve as the most popular determining factors to assess credibility of health information among young people, keep in mind that there are legitimate Internet sites, databases, and books that publish health information and serve as sources of health information for doctors, other health sites, and members of the public. For example, MedlinePlus (https://medlineplus.gov) has trusted sources on over 975 diseases and conditions and presents the information in easy-to-understand language.

The chart here presents factors to consider when assessing credibility of health information. However, keep in mind that these factors function only as a guide and require continuous updating to keep abreast with the changes in the landscape of health information, information sources, and technologies.

The chart can serve as a guide; however, approaching a librarian about how one can go about assessing the credibility of both print and online health information is far more effective than using generic checklist-type

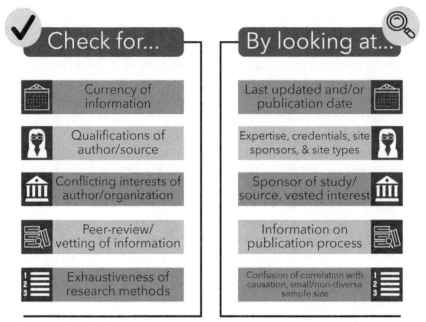

All images from flaticon.com

tools. While librarians are not health experts, they can apply and teach patrons strategies to determine the credibility of health information.

With the prevalence of fake sites and fake resources that appear to be legitimate, it is important to use the following health information assessment tips to verify health information that one has obtained (St. Jean et al., 2015, p. 151):

- **Don't assume you are right**: Even when you feel very sure about an answer, keep in mind that the answer may not be correct, and it is important to conduct (further) searches to validate the information.
- **Don't assume you are wrong**: You may actually have correct information, even if the information you encounter does not match—that is, you may be right and the resources that you have found may contain false information.
- **Take an open approach**: Maintain a critical stance by not including your preexisting beliefs as keywords (or letting them influence your choice of keywords) in a search, as this may influence what it is possible to find out.
- **Verify, verify, and verify**: Information found, especially on the Internet, needs to be validated, no matter how the information appears on

the site (i.e., regardless of the appearance of the site or the quantity of information that is included).

Health literacy comes with experience navigating health information. Professional sources of health information, such as doctors, health-care providers, and health databases, are still the best, but one also has the power to search for health information and then verify it by consulting with these trusted sources and by using the health information assessment tips and guide shared previously.

Mega Subramaniam, PhD
Associate Professor, College of Information Studies,
University of Maryland

REFERENCES AND FURTHER READING

American Association of School Librarians (AASL). (2009). *Standards for the 21st-century learner in action.* Chicago, IL: American Association of School Librarians.

Hilligoss, B., & Rieh, S.-Y. (2008). Developing a unifying framework of credibility assessment: Construct, heuristics, and interaction in context. *Information Processing & Management, 44*(4), 1467–1484.

Kuhlthau, C. C. (1988). Developing a model of the library search process: Cognitive and affective aspects. *Reference Quarterly, 28*(2), 232–242.

National Network of Libraries of Medicine (NNLM). (2013). Health literacy. Bethesda, MD: National Network of Libraries of Medicine. Retrieved from nnlm.gov/outreach/consumer/hlthlit.html

Ratzan, S. C., & Parker, R. M. (2000). Introduction. In C. R. Selden, M. Zorn, S. C. Ratzan, & R. M. Parker (Eds.), *National Library of Medicine current bibliographies in medicine: Health literacy.* NLM Pub. No. CBM 2000-1. Bethesda, MD: National Institutes of Health, U.S. Department of Health and Human Services.

St. Jean, B., Taylor, N. G., Kodama, C., & Subramaniam, M. (February 2017). Assessing the health information source perceptions of tweens using card-sorting exercises. *Journal of Information Science.* Retrieved from http://journals.sagepub.com/doi/abs/10.1177/0165551516687728

St. Jean, B., Subramaniam, M., Taylor, N. G., Follman, R., Kodama, C., & Casciotti, D. (2015). The influence of positive hypothesis testing on youths' online health-related information seeking. *New Library World, 116*(3/4), 136–154.

Subramaniam, M., St. Jean, B., Taylor, N. G., Kodama, C., Follman, R., & Casciotti, D. (2015). Bit by bit: Using design-based research to improve the health literacy of adolescents. *JMIR Research Protocols*, 4(2), paper e62. Retrieved from http://www.ncbi.nlm.nih.gov/pmc /articles/PMC4464334/

Valenza, J. (2016, November 26). Truth, truthiness, and triangulation: A news literacy toolkit for a "post-truth" world [Web log]. Retrieved from http://blogs.slj.com/neverendingsearch/2016/11/26/truth-truthi ness-triangulation-and-the-librarian-way-a-news-literacy-toolkit-for -a-post-truth-world/

Common Misconceptions about Sport Injuries

1. THERE IS NO GAIN WITHOUT PAIN

Today, the importance of regular physical activity as a way to promote health and wellness is undeniable. One prevailing idea is that if exercise is good for you, then more exercise must be better. Exercise should hurt. The phrase "No gain without pain" has been around for some time, but it was actress Jane Fonda who capitalized on this through a popular television show and her best-selling workout videos. "No gain without pain" is a clever saying, but if it is your catchphrase, you are setting yourself up for failure either by quitting or by injury. Discomfort and pain are not the same. Let's say you have been using swimming as your exercise program for the summer but have now returned to the gym. You start doing squats again. You feel fatigue in your quadriceps (the big thigh muscles). The muscles might feel a little full and tight, and you are a little uncomfortable. You may actually feel a little burning when you do the squats, but that goes away within a minute after completing the exercise. You're a little tired, and the next day you experience some soreness. This is a normal response to an unfamiliar exercise. But if you experience a short pain in the knee, hip, or back, then this is not normal. The pain is a symptom of tissue damage, and you should stop. Some athletes suggest working through the pain, but this is a terrible idea, causing even more damage.

That's not the answer. Pain indicates injury, and you need to respect the body's signals. Pain is our indicator that something is wrong. To learn more about exercise intensity, see Question 37.

2. INCREASING FLEXIBILITY WILL DECREASE THE FREQUENCY OF INJURY

It seems somewhat reasonable to surmise that if a body part is stretched beyond its normal limits, increased flexibility might reduce injury. This idea supports the training goal of increased flexibility. Interestingly, video analyses of injury indicate that most musculoskeletal injuries occur within the normal range of motion (ROM), making one question whether it is necessary to increase flexibility. What is the normal ROM? Even a casual observer might note that some sports require far more flexibility than others. A normal ROM for one athlete is not normal for others. Gymnasts, ballet dancers, figure skaters, and divers require a ROM much greater than soccer or basketball players. Each sport has a specific normal ROM. Studies have shown that increasing the flexibility of athletes beyond what is required in sport does not reduce the incidence of injury. Are flexible joints actually more susceptible to injury? Athletes must be able to move comfortably throughout their ROM. Training for flexibility should include static and dynamic stretching activities designed to improve and maintain the ROM required by their sport. Pre-event static stretching is not recommended for some activities. To learn more about flexibility training and pre-event stretching, see Question 42.

3. A CONCUSSION ONLY OCCURS WHEN THERE IS A LOSS OF CONSCIOUSNESS

Concussions have become an important topic of conversation recently, primarily because of the long-term effects suffered by many well-known professional football players. In extreme circumstances, the long-term effect of repeated concussions on players' brains has actually led them to commit suicide. Concussions are not limited to football players. Almost any athlete can experience one. You can get a concussion diving into the pool, not by hitting the board but by hitting the water. Participants in dodge ball get concussions. Concussions can be treated successfully, but treatment requires that the concussion be identified. Doctors often call a concussion a mild brain injury, not because it is not serious but because a single concussion is usually not life-threatening. Diagnosis is so important because a subsequent concussion before recovery can be lethal.

The second concussion can lead to secondary impact syndrome, serious swelling of the brain that can lead to severe disability or death. One misconception about diagnosis is that a concussion is accompanied by unconsciousness. The person is "knocked out." The Centers for Disease Control has pointed out that most concussions do not result in unconsciousness. Studies have shown that most athletes are unaware of the symptoms of concussion. To understand more about concussion symptoms and treatment, see Questions 16 and 28.

4. WHEN PAIN IS GONE, YOU ARE READY TO RETURN TO COMPETITION

When athletes are injured, one of the first questions asked is when can they return to play. The athlete wants to play, and the coach and team need them. There's a lot of pressure to return. Most sports are seasonal, and seasons end; there are only so many games to play, and athletes want to experience all of them. When an injury occurs, the body goes through well-established stages of healing. Each of these stages takes time. Although therapy can reduce the time, if the same injury occurs prior to recovery, the length of time needed to heal is increased. Reinjury takes longer. Furthermore, returning to play too early can place other parts of the body in jeopardy. A compromised joint or muscle can change well-established movement patterns, resulting in excessive stress on other parts of the movement chain. When to return to play is always a tricky business. Athletes often believe that when pain is gone, they are ready to return. Pain-free ROM is extremely important in the rehabilitation phase of injury, but it is not the criterion for return to play. The functional ability of the athlete is the primary criterion. Is the athlete prepared to play at full speed? Can the athlete meet the demands of the sport? Since fatigue is related to injury, has the athlete trained enough so that they are not unduly fatigued? To learn more about the stages of injury and return-to-play guidelines, see Questions 9 and 35.

5. SURGERY WILL MAKE YOU GOOD AS NEW

Modern humans have been around for around 200,000 years, having evolved for several million years. This evolution has resulted in a marvelous body capable of withstanding enormous stress and temperature with the ability to adapt. We have a neuromuscular system capable of intricate as well as powerful movements, a skeletal structure that is the marvel of engineering, and the most powerful brain of all animals. Surgery may fix acute problems but cannot overcome the effects of evolution. Fortunately, surgery is not as invasive as it once was. The advent of arthroscopic surgery and other less invasive tools for surgery have reduced recovery time and damage. But surgery is still invasive, requiring an entrance into our bodies that will always leave a mark. Surgery can relieve pain, such as by setting a broken bone. Surgery on a torn muscle or ligament leaves compromised tissue. A joint injury that requires surgery leaves a joint that is always compromised. Surgeries fix problems, but the end result has long-lasting impact. Many of these problems eventually cause osteoarthritis, a common condition that affects us as we age. Surgery is often necessary, but it won't make us good as new. To learn more about surgery for sport injuries, see Question 32.

QUESTIONS AND ANSWERS

The Basics

1. What are sport injuries?

A sport injury is any injury incurred as a result of participation in a sport or exercise. When we think of sport injuries, we often think of football or ice hockey, but people get hurt playing tennis or golf, riding horseback, cycling, cheerleading, or doing yoga poses. Fortunately, most sport injuries are not serious, and a few days' rest returns one to form. Injuries to the musculoskeletal system are the most common sport injuries, but participants can also receive an injury to the nervous system. Sport injuries can be psychological and can result in behaviors that are detrimental to participants as well as friends and family.

Injuries to the musculoskeletal system remain the most common form of sport injury. A review of the literature generally lists the following as the most common sport injuries:

1. Strains—hamstring, quadriceps, hip flexors, and groin injuries
2. Sprains—ankle, knee
3. Knee injuries—anterior cruciate ligament (ACL) tears, meniscus tears, patella femoral
4. Fractures—clavicle (collar bone), fibula (outer bone in lower leg)
5. Tennis elbow
6. Shin splints

7. Back pain/injury
8. Concussion

Participants in sport frequently get cuts, bruises, and blisters; lose teeth; and dislocate shoulders, although not as frequent as the preceding injuries. Participants are far more likely to injure their lower body than their upper extremities. All of these injuries can range from a fairly simple disruption to one that sidelines the person for a year, or even a lifetime. For example, while these both are labeled as muscle strains, a muscle strain can range from a mild tear of a few small fibers to the total disruption of the muscle from the bone, requiring surgery to reattach the muscle. A lost tooth in high school requires a lifetime of dentures.

Injuries to the nervous system are not common and normally involve peripheral nerves. Your peripheral nerves are the links between your brain and spinal cord and the rest of your body. A nerve injury can affect your brain's ability to communicate with your muscles and organs, the primary reason that individuals may feel numbness in their extremity. Peripheral nerves are fragile and easily damaged usually by compression (a blow) or being stretched. The most common of these nerve injuries is the "burner," mostly observed in football players and wrestlers. This injury is often the result of a severe twisting of the head or shoulder and causes a burning sensation, a condition that resolves in a few minutes.

Sport injuries are more than musculoskeletal or nerve problems; they can be psychological as well. Exercise addiction has become a label linked to those obsessed with exercise. People with exercise addiction tend to increase their tolerance; suffer withdrawal when not exercising; and spend a great deal of time preparing for, engaging in, and recovering from exercise. Exercise rules their lives. People with body image problems (body dysmorphia), low self-esteem, and lack of confidence seem more at risk. Exercise addiction can also be associated with an eating disorder. Regardless of the reason, exercise addiction can wreak havoc on a person's life as well as their family and friends. Furthermore, individuals with exercise addiction tend to exercise even when injured, further exacerbating the initial injury. It is estimated that about 3 percent of the exercising public develop exercise addiction.

Almost everyone from the average gym participant to the athlete in training will likely suffer a sport injury, whether physical or mental. An injury is one of the primary reasons that individuals quit their exercise routine. Fortunately, most sport injuries are not serious, quickly heal, and have no lifetime effects.

2. How common are sport injuries, and who gets them?

Everyone is susceptible to a sport injury. Whether you exercise to maintain or improve fitness, play a recreational sport, or compete on a high school or college team, you will probably have to confront a sport injury. No one is immune from a sport injury, regardless of age, experience, or fitness. Sport injuries are painful, may require you to miss work or school, and are detrimental to your quality of life. Anyone who chooses to participate in sport or exercise should learn how to train so that they enjoy the benefits of exercise while reducing the chance of injury. Although people who exercise risk injury, the rewards of regular exercise far outweigh the risk of leading a sedentary lifestyle.

Competitive sports, because of their increased intensity, result in the most sport injuries. Athletes in competitive sports now tend to play just one sport all year. Some years back, athletes in high school played two or three sports a year, thus allowing the athlete to rest muscle groups as the pattern of sport changed. Playing the same sport all year causes more muscle and tendon fatigue than seasonal play; fatigue leads to injury. Individuals playing contact sports like football, men's lacrosse, and ice hockey are particularly affected. Women gymnasts and soccer players are much more likely to be injured than women swimmers. The National Collegiate Athletic Association maintains injury statistics for 25 men and women's collegiate sports. For men, football, followed by wrestling and ice hockey, has the highest rate of injury. For women, soccer has the highest rate of injury, with gymnastics and ice hockey almost as risky. Data show that high school athletes follow a similar pattern of injury.

Is gender a factor in competitive sports? The overall risk of injury for men is higher, but it is mainly because of men's football and wrestling. In general, the risk of injury for men and women is similar, but with small differences. For example, women's soccer has a greater risk than men's soccer, but men's basketball has a higher risk than women's basketball. In regard to the type of injuries, the most startling difference is the higher rate of knee injury for women.

Studies have shown that women tend to injure their knees two to eight times more frequently than men. Injury to the anterior cruciate ligament (ACL), the small ligament that attaches the front of the tibia to the back of the femur, is problematic. Many knee injuries do not require surgery, but ACL tears routinely end up being surgically repaired. Furthermore, ACL surgery requires about one year of intense rehabilitation before the individual can return to competition; some never return. ACL injuries frequently occur when athletes land, stop, or turn quickly. Studies have found that women's landing and turning mechanics are not as protective as men's; the muscles that contract to absorb shock contract more slowly. The rationale for this difference has not been determined, but many suggest that boys spend more time playing sports when they are young than girls, thereby developing proper muscle recruitment early in life. Programs to improve landing mechanics to reduce the frequency of knee injuries have proved effective. See Question 47 for more information.

Millions of individuals in the United States play sports in a recreational fashion, while others work to improve their fitness. Interestingly, participation in fitness activities has not always been common. Jogging didn't start until 1968, following the publication of Ken Cooper's best-selling book, *Aerobics*. Cooper's book was the beginning of the fitness revolution that is still in existence today. After 1968, we saw runners everywhere—old, young, men, and women. To meet this interest, fitness centers for adults were built everywhere; exercise programs for young and old were touted; and exercise was for sale. Unfortunately, many of the individuals selling exercise were not trained.

After 1968, sport injuries became commonplace. The stress and strain of exercise on the unfit public led to an increased number of sport injuries. Overweight individuals turned to exercise as a way to lose weight, leading to excess stress on knees, hips, and backs. People with pronated feet, hyperextending knees, or poor form chose activities unsuitable for them. A common question in exercise has always been, "How much exercise is enough?" Motivated participants would inevitably do too much too soon, not giving time for their bodies to adapt to the training. Overuse injuries became common, almost unheard of prior to 1968; even children were getting overuse injuries.

Although sport injuries are common, the frequency of injury in many sports is not that high. Question 5 addresses the question of injury incidence in various activities. Meanwhile, of all the factors related to injury frequency, prior injury is the most significant predictor; injuries tend to recur. Recidivism (the tendency to recur) happens for two reasons: (1) the injured individual returns to exercise or play before they have fully recovered, or (2) the individual has a biomechanical structure that places undue stress on a body part.

3. What is the cost of sport injuries?

Each year about 30 million children play some form of organized sport. About 10 percent of these will suffer some form of injury that will require medical treatment. About 8 million boys and girls play interscholastic sport, resulting in around 2 million injuries and 30,000 hospitalizations. The cost of contact sports per year in college ranged from $446 million to $1.5 billion; for high school, the range was $5.4–$19.2 billion. These are the short-term costs with no accounting for future costs. Additionally, millions of adults exercise on a regular basis, accounting for several million injuries and untold expense. The cost of all of these injuries is astronomical. Unfortunately, many individuals who do get injured are uninsured. Not only do uninsured individuals have to pay out of pocket, but they also may pay more, since they do not have the support of an insurance company that sets prices.

Predicting the cost of all of these injuries is virtually impossible for a number of reasons. First, the range of charges at different hospitals is wide. Second, many injuries result in absence from work or school. An injury may require you to drop out of school or quit work. The cost of this loss is unaccountable. Third, an early injury during youth may result in an expensive surgery 30 years later. For example, early knee injuries may eventually result in a $55,000 knee replacement. Fourth, you cannot put a monetary value on something that negatively impacts your life. For instance, what if you love downhill skiing, but a serious knee injury playing basketball makes skiing uncomfortable? Skiing is not as fun. You can fall off your bike and dislocate your shoulder, and your tennis game is now problematic. Overhead serves hurt. Tennis isn't as fun as it used to be. All in all, the real cost of sport injuries is astounding.

A major factor in the cost of a sport injury is whether you are treated in the emergency room (ER). The primary injuries presented at ERs are a sprain or a strain. Nationwide, the average ER cost for these injuries is about $1,233, but one study indicated costs over $20,000. Presumably these extra costs are for extensive tests prescribed by orthopedic specialists. A recent alternative to the ER is an urgent care center (UCC). Not all cities have an UCC, but the average cost for visiting a UCC is $150. Many small injuries can be treated well in an ER, but if there is any life-threatening injury, the ER in a hospital is the definite choice. Table 1 presents some of the typical costs for injuries. Keep in mind that these are average figures and that the range is wide.

A study conducted by a physicians group in San Francisco found that 32 percent of patients visiting the ER for sprains and strains were uninsured. To reduce cost, the study suggested that individuals should develop a relationship with a medical doctor who can help navigate the unlikely event that one needs to go to the ER. A second suggestion was to have a physician who is available enough that the ER is not the only option.

Table 1 Average Cost of Treatment Nationwide

Treatment	Average Cost
Leg fracture	$3,400
Arm fracture	$7,600
Dislocation (shoulder)	$4,600
Concussion	$1,000–$7,000*
Stitches (ER)	$500/stitch
Stitches (UCC)	$150–$300
Tooth replacement (implant)	$4,200
Ambulance	$225–$2,200
Physical therapy treatment	$150

*Prices vary widely for concussion treatment—some sources indicate $18,454.

Finally, having some kind of catastrophic (but cheaper) insurance can keep you from bankruptcy.

Sport injuries occasionally require surgery. One of the most common surgeries is arthroscopic surgery to the knee to repair the meniscus (meniscectomy). Prior to the arthroscope, these surgeries were only done in hospitals and required multiple days of hospital care. Today, most of these surgeries do not require any hospitalization, and patients can usually walk with some support within a day or two. The cost of this surgery varies with whether it is conducted in an inpatient hospital versus an outpatient hospital. Many large orthopedic practices have their own operating facility that is strictly outpatient. You arrive in the morning, and someone drives you home later in the day after you recover. The average price for knee surgery in these facilities is $12,500, while a full service hospital will charge around $21,990 for the same surgery.

4. Can sport injuries have lifelong effects?

When people are injured while pursuing sports and fitness, the first question most asked is, How long before I can get back to my activity? The long-term effect is rarely considered, but many sport injuries have effects that can last a lifetime. This doesn't mean that every injury will present long-term problems. When most people get injured, they get care, rest, and return to play. Cuts, bruises, soreness, and many small sprains heal and go away. When a child athlete breaks an arm or leg, it quickly heals, and there are no aftereffects. The fact that some injuries have lasting effects is not a reason to stay away from sports and fitness. Millions of people play many sports, don't get injured, and have a normal life.

However, injuries can have negative effects throughout life if not taken care of properly. Athletes sometimes push themselves despite the severity of an injury, driving themselves to play even when hurt. There is pressure to return early from an injury, a practice that often results in a more severe injury. Acute sprains, such as an ankle, can turn into a permanent unstable ankle. Patella and shoulder dislocations, tennis elbow, and low back pain can all become lifelong problems if not allowed to recover completely.

The most debilitating problem for older adults is osteoarthritis (OA). Most adults in their fifties have some form of mild OA, and some develop OA symptoms that are quite painful, affecting quality of life and work habits and occasionally resulting in joint replacement. OA is a disease of joints and is associated with the layer of cartilage that covers each bone in the body. The purpose of this articular (joint) cartilage is to protect the ends of bones, to displace some of the stress on joints. If and when the articular cartilage degenerates, the bone is unprotected; pain and a loss of motion are the result. This loss of articular cartilage results in OA. Sports that subject the individual to high levels of torsional (twisting) stress increase the degeneration of articular cartilage.

The knee joint is clearly the most common OA site. A common injury in many sports, especially football, basketball, and soccer, is a torn meniscus. Because the knee undergoes such tremendous stress, extra cushioning is provided by two articulating disks (menisci) attached to the top of the tibia (shin bone). But these menisci can be torn by increased torsion during intense exercise. Removal of the torn meniscus (meniscectomy) is reasonably simple and effective, but the lack of extra cushioning leaves the joint cartilage more vulnerable to wear and tear; the result is often OA. A torn meniscus often accompanies a more serious knee injury, rupture of the anterior cruciate ligament (ACL). About 50 percent of athletes who have a ruptured ACL/meniscus tear develop OA within 10–20 years.

Evidence suggests that there is no harmful effect on joints for individuals pursuing moderate recreational activity and having normal joint activity. Runners often ask whether jogging causes OA. Individuals who have no joint abnormalities often experience a lifetime of jogging without developing OA. However, this is not the case for individuals who have had a meniscectomy; removing part of the meniscus is a harbinger of knee problems for joggers. There does seem to be an association between elite sports participation and an increased risk of OA, especially in those sports involving high-intensity, high-impact forces and especially where the injury rate is high such as football and ice hockey.

One injury that can result in serious longstanding effects is a concussion. Concussions do not have to have lifelong effects; in fact, most people who receive a concussion have no long-term problems. But while a number of effects such as headaches, light sensitivity, and vertigo can last a year or more following a concussion, lifelong effects are more serious. In recent years, there has been considerable publicity involving NFL football players who have often suffered many concussions. The effects on some of these players have been so severe that they have committed suicide. Chronic traumatic encephalopathy (CTE), a degenerative brain disease, is often the culprit. Concussions are the chief cause of CTE, although it is unlikely that a single concussive injury brings on CTE. Symptoms tend to show about 15 years after one's career ends and includes the following:

- Cognitive impairment, such as memory loss
- Speech and language difficulties
- Depression and aggression
- Dementia

Long-term problems from concussions are not relegated to professional football players. Participants in basketball, soccer, ice hockey, and lacrosse can suffer concussions. High school football players get concussions. Publicity has changed the way coaches, athletic trainers, and the public have viewed concussions in youth and collegiate sport. Today, blows to the head that might cause a concussion are treated seriously.

Can sport injuries to children lead to lifelong problems? As more and more children participate in organized sport, one concern is the possible prolonged effect of injury to children. Normally, children get hurt, get treatment, and return to sport when they are healed. There are no long-term negative effects. One major concern is whether an injury can affect growth. At each end of long bones, there is a growth center, the epiphysis. When an injury such as a broken bone occurs at the growth center of the bone, there is the concern that uneven growth may occur. These injuries require proper care by a physician followed by complete recovery.

Once injured, is it possible to reduce the risk of negative long-term effects? Many athletes finish their athletic careers faced with the possibility of a lifetime of physical problems. Concern is warranted as research has shown the increased risk of problems deriving from early injuries. Since the beneficial effects of regular exercise are well accepted, most individuals wish to maintain an active lifestyle. Fortunately, research has shown that regular exercise has a positive impact on OA. The answer is to exercise in a way that does not exacerbate the original problem. Additionally, putting oneself at risk of experiencing the same injury should be avoided.

With regard to concussions, it is clear that avoiding additional head injury is mandated. Group sports like touch football and soccer should be avoided. Do not do any headfirst dives off high places. Ice or roller skating is not a good idea. If living in a cold climate with ice on sidewalks and driveways, wear some form of traction device on shoes or boots. Wear a well-designed helmet when skiing and biking. It is possible to reduce possible lifelong consequences, but these adaptations to lifestyle require a change in behavior and an awareness that continued damage will result otherwise.

5. Are certain sports more or less likely to lead to injury?

As reported in Questions 1 and 2, people encounter sport injuries in many activities from those individuals participating in school-sponsored competitive sports to those just working out or playing a recreational sport like tennis or softball. Competitive sports, because of their increased intensity and lengthy season, clearly result in the most sport injuries across the country. Unlike most recreational sports and activities, many competitive sports like football and ice hockey also involve bodily contact. Participants in recreational sports suffer their share of injuries and fitness participants who jog, cycle, and lift weights also get hurt.

The National Collegiate Athletic Association (NCAA) and many interscholastic organizations keep data on the frequency and types of injury. When observing this data, it is important to understand that there is a difference in the number of injuries compared with the rate of injury. For example, women's basketball results in far more injuries than women's gymnastics, but the rate of injury in gymnastics is much higher; gymnasts are more likely to get injured than basketball players. Table 2 provides data on the injury rate for many competitive sports.

Men's football accounts for the most college sport injuries (31 percent of all male injuries) and the highest rate of more serious injuries requiring more than seven days to return to practice (26.2 percent), surgery (40.2 percent), and injuries requiring emergency transportation (31.9 percent). The rate of injury during football competition is very high compared to other sports (40 injuries per 1,000 exposures). Women's soccer clearly

Table 2 Injury Rate by Sport in Competitive Athletics

	Men's Sports	Women's Sports
Highest rate of injury	Football	Soccer
	Wrestling	Gymnastics
	Ice hockey	Ice hockey
	Soccer	Field hockey
	Basketball	Basketball
	Lacrosse	Lacrosse
	Tennis	Cross country
	Basketball	Tennis
	Indoor track	Volleyball
	Outdoor track	Softball
	Cross country	Outdoor track
Lowest rate of injury	Swimming and diving	Swimming and diving

accounts for the most injuries per year for women. Women's soccer also has a rather high injury rate during competition (17.2 injuries per 1,000 exposures).

Competitive athletes encounter injuries both in practice and competition, but the injury rate in competition is far higher than in practice. However, athletes practice four to five times more during practice than during competition; the total number of injuries is about the same for practice and competition. Athletes are far more likely to get injured during the preseason. Coaches are commonly in a rush to get their athletes ready for competition, and practices are generally longer. Further, many athletes are not fit for the rigors of practice, suffer extensive fatigue, and get hurt. Also, sports like football, soccer, and field hockey often start at the end of summer when it is still hot and humid. Not only do these athletes have to contend with intense training, but they also must battle the heat and humidity. Dehydration and hyperthermia prevail.

Cheerleading can be a dangerous sport. Injury rate in cheerleading is somewhat vague since there are no mandatory reporting systems for most cheerleaders. Some cheerleading teams are under the auspices of the Athletic Department, while some are not. Some may not think of cheerleading as a sport, but cheerleaders have summer camps, tryouts, and regular practice, and many have competitions. Most people think of cheering as the groups leading cheers on the sidelines of football and basketball games, but cheerleading has changed into a very competitive activity with many gymnastic maneuvers and pyramids. Injury rate in cheerleading is similar to most sports with ankle sprains being the most frequent injury. Unlike most sports, cheerleaders encounter a number of neck and low back sprains as a result of gymnastic-like activities. Catastrophic injuries are one of the major problems with cheerleading, as 70.5 percent of all college catastrophic injuries to female athletes occur in cheerleading; high school athletes face a similar problem, with 65.2 percent of catastrophic injuries. Catastrophic injuries are skull fractures, cervical fractures, and occasional deaths. Most catastrophic injuries happen during practice when athletes are performing high-risk stunts like pyramids.

While football players may have the highest number of sport injuries for competitive sports, cycling has the highest absolute number of injuries of all activities (614,594). Cycling is enjoyed by people of all ages, as they bike for transportation, cycle for exercise, or race. In recent years, road cycling as a sport and recreational activity has increased. Bicycle injuries can be acute or overuse. Traumatic injuries include collision with another rider or a vehicle. Most of these are to the upper body, the head, or the collarbone or shoulder. Acute injuries are generally abrasions. One study (reported in the *International Journal of Sports Medicine*) followed 512 recreational riders for a year and found that 85 percent reported one or more chronic overuse injuries in one year. The knee clearly suffers the most overuse injuries followed by the wrist. Most overuse injuries are not real serious, and a week off the bike is usually all one needs.

Mountain biking (also called off-road biking) is no longer a minor biking subcategory, but it is the fastest area of growth in cycling in the last 20 years. Mountain bikes account for more sales than any other category of bicycle. Mountain bikers do not usually have overuse injuries and are not involved with vehicular contact. The overall injury rate for mountain bikers is higher than for road bikers, but the injuries are generally minimal, involving scrapes and lacerations. Most of these can be self-treated and do not involve hospitalization. The overall risk of mountain biking is similar to road biking. Poor judgment accounts for about 90 percent of mountain bike injuries, including excessive speed (36 percent), unfamiliar terrain (35 percent), inattention (23 percent), and riding beyond one's level (20 percent).

Running continues to be one of the most popular aerobic exercises across the country. Almost 30 million Americans participate in a regular running program. Many runners enjoy the benefits of running; little equipment is necessary, and one can run alone most anywhere, anytime.

The injury rate is reported to be somewhere between 37 and 57 percent per year. Recreational runners tend to be at the lower end of the range; the rate is higher for competitive runners. The knee is the most common injury site, accounting for 30–50 percent of all injuries. The lower leg and foot are also common injury sites. Running injuries are more related to overuse, and most are the result of training errors, such as an abrupt increase in mileage, too much high-intensity training without rest, excessive hill running, and surface changes.

Racket sports are one of the more popular recreational sports, with tennis clearly leading the list over squash, badminton, and racquetball. Compared to most sports, the injury rate is relatively low with a reported incidence varying from 0.04 injuries/1,000 hours to 3.0 injuries/1,000 hours. The most common acute injuries happen to the ankle and knee (patella tendonitis), while overuse injuries occur in the shoulder, elbow, and wrist. Low back and spine injuries also occur. Factors that may affect injury rate are the playing surface and playing duration. The injury rate increases for those playing more than two hours a session.

Weight training and calisthenic (body weight) exercises are very common among fitness participants. Recreational weight training has a relatively low injury rate, but individuals who do a lot of overhead work, such as in Olympic lifts, have more low back and shoulder problems. Extensive high-intensity exercises while the spine is flexed tend to result in more back problems. Calisthenic exercises are generally safe, but participants need to understand that doing the exact routine day after day can result in overuse; mixing up activities should be considered. In the past few years, there has been excessive focus on developing distinctive abdominal muscles (the so-called six pack). Extensive sit-ups and other abdominal exercises place a lot of stress on the lumbar spine causing low back pain.

The more you exercise and play, the greater chance you have of getting hurt. For example, running, biking, and tennis are relatively safe exercises, but when the activity becomes excessive, the injury rate goes up. Weight training is generally safe, but this can be overdone as well. One group that occasionally leads to excessive exercise is CrossFit. CrossFit's unofficial mascot is Rhabdo, short for rhabdomyolysis, a serious condition related to significant muscle damage. Normally, rhabdomyolysis is caused by muscle trauma, but exercisers (particularly novices) are sometimes encouraged to push themselves so hard that there is excessive muscle damage. The kidneys cannot clear the damaged tissue and tend to fail. Most people who experience rhabdomyolysis have significant swelling and discomfort in their muscles, but some individuals have actually died from excessive muscle damage. Sport and activity is generally safe, but if the exercise is disproportionate and rest is inadequate, injury usually follows.

6. Who is a weekend warrior? Why is being one a problem?

Lack of time is the primary reason cited for not regularly exercising. According to a national Gallup poll, the average American worker works 47 hours a week, or 9.4 hours a day, while many say they work 50 hours a week or more. In the United States, 86 percent of males and 67 percent of females work more than 40 hours a week. Americans work more now than some years back, and surveys indicate that Americans work more than any other industrialized country. Meanwhile, there's no denying the benefits of exercise. So what is a person supposed to do? Weekend warriors are often the resort. Some have defined weekend warriors as an individual who does not have time to exercise during the week and pushes all of their recreational activities and exercise into two days a week.

As presented throughout this text and especially in the section on injury prevention, the incidence of a sport injury can be reduced by being physically prepared for whatever activity in which one engages. Even then, participants get hurt. The true weekend warrior actually has five days between activities, a time when many of the training adaptations are lost. Furthermore, some sources suggest that weekend warriors compensate by choosing physically strenuous activities on the weekend. Subsequently, weekend warriors are at significant risk of injury because of their lack of preparation and exercise intensity.

Emergency room (ER) physicians are well aware when the recreational softball season starts. A quick look down the gurneys in the ER often show a row of softball cleats attached to weekend warriors with muscle strains and sprains and the occasional broken arm or ankle. Sports like softball, touch football, and pickup basketball require athletes to recruit muscle fibers they do not train even if they do prepare. Let's say you get up to bat, hit the ball, and sprint to first base to beat out the throw. You catch a ball in the outfield and throw home as hard as you can to catch the incoming runner. How about sliding into second? How did you prepare for that? What about jumping for a rebound in basketball? Even though a weekend warrior may find some time to do some preparation like jogging or some floor exercises, they are not prepared for the intensity of competition exhibited in a game that requires high-intensity muscle contractions.

Sprinting, high-velocity throwing, and jumping recruit one's fast-twitch muscle fibers. The muscles in our body are composed of a combination of slow- and fast-twitch fibers. Activities like jogging, playing catch, and many floor exercises only recruit slow-twitch fibers. Sprinting, high-speed throwing, and jumping recruit the more powerful fast-twitch fibers. Even though activities like jogging and throwing use the same muscle groups, the individual fibers within the muscle are not prepared unless you train these specific fibers.

The primary sport injuries for weekend warriors are strains and sprains to the lower body. Strained hamstrings, high flexors, and groin muscles are the common strains, while knee and ankle sprains are the common sprains. Let's say you have signed up for a softball or basketball league that plays on the weekend. Try to get in some playing time prior to the start of competition, but take the time to adapt. Fortunately, there are some activities one can do at home that will help reduce the frequency of injury. These are activities that engage your fast-twitch fibers but only if done correctly and with rest intervals. Fast-twitch fibers are anaerobic (not endurance) fibers, so rest intervals are required. The following activities will help, but remember to precede these by warming up with lower intensity activities:

- Vertical jumping—jump as high as you can and touch the wall
- Jump as high as you can and land on one foot—maintain your balance
- Split jumps—from a split-stance position, jump into the air and switch legs on landing
- Horizontal jumps—leap forward three to four times but jump as soon as you land
- Single-leg hops—hop on one foot four to five times, then use both feet; stop after each and maintain balance
- Bounding—run three to four steps and then hop three to four times on one foot
- Side hops—put three books on floor, hop sideways over each one on one foot, switch feet, and hop back three to four times
- Skipping—skip vigorously on the sidewalk or backyard
- Stair running—run up a flight of stairs preceded by a short run; use every second or third step
- Sprints—sprint 20 yards preceded by warm-up
- Ball throws—use a tennis ball and slowly increase throwing velocity against a wall

Some of these activities are more difficult. For example, bounding on one foot is quite strenuous, so do not start off with this activity. Sprinting requires a warm-up and a progression of several weeks. Fortunately, doing these activities will also make you more powerful. Finally, warming up prior to play is particularly important for weekend warriors. A week of sitting at a desk is going to make you stiff, so a proper warm-up is essential. Arrive at the game or activity early to give you time. Feel free to do some stretching, but remember that only dynamic muscle contractions will warm up muscles and joints.

7. Does specializing in a sport increase the likelihood of injury?

For generations, children played sports informally, organizing and officiating themselves and playing seasonally, and eventually joined interscholastic school teams as they got older. Meanwhile, professional athletes began amassing fortunes as a result of their success on the playing fields or in the gym. Colleges placed more emphasis on sport, and high school athletes were recruited to play at the nation's top universities. Athletic success was a way to achieve the American dream. Parents, wishing to give their children the best life possible, adopted the idea that an early, intense start in sport was one key to athletic success. Sport specialization, intense, year-round training in a single sport with the exclusion of other sport, became common practice for many. With regard to sport specialization, two questions are generally asked: Does specializing in one sport at a young age develop better athletes? and does specializing in one sport increase the likelihood of injury?

Although the focus of this text is sport injury, the answer to the first question is that it is not necessary to specialize in sport at an early age to achieve top-level success. Numerous studies by the Canadian Institute of Sport for Life have shown that sampling multiple sports does not compromise athletic success. Most top-level athletes did not specialize in youth. Pete Carroll, former football coach of the University of Southern California, said, "The first question I ask is, 'What other sports does he play' . . . I really, really don't favor kids who specialize in one sport." Even in a non–team sport like tennis, Roger Federer played multiple sports in youth until finally specializing in tennis.

Regarding sport injuries for those who specialize, there are two problems: injury and burnout. For many years, acute injuries, such as a sprained ankle or wrist, were the predominant injury among children. But as children began to train more in a single sport, they began to incur overuse injuries. Overuse injuries occur due to repetitive submaximal loading of the musculoskeletal system accompanied by inadequate rest. This has become particularly common among youth who specialize, since they engage in the same movements repeatedly. Overuse injury involves the muscle, tendon, bone, and growth centers.

One issue with youth sport is that the children are growing while training. Furthermore, growth is not linear. For example, muscles attach via tendon to bones. In Question 5, epiphysis was discussed as the growth center of bones. In addition to this primary epiphysis, there are secondary epiphyses that develop where muscles are pulling on bones. Small bumps (tuberosities) on the bone are created to improve the leverage of muscle pull, but the bone may not develop as fast as the muscle attached to it. Significant muscle development through training may disrupt the site of tendon/bone connection, causing Osgood-Schlatter's disease (knee) or Sever's disease (heel). These injuries, called apophyseal injuries, are unique to youth.

There have not been sufficient studies on the relationship between sport specialization and the frequency of injury. However, the limited studies to date suggest that those who specialize, especially those who specialized the most, were 81 percent more likely to suffer an overuse injury compared to those who played a wide variety of sports. The youth who specialized the most identified a primary sport, trained more than eight months/year, and quit all other sports. It seems clear that sport specialization results in an increased incidence of injury.

For many years, youth baseball pitchers were at increased risk of shoulder and elbow injury. Little League coaches had their good pitchers pitch many games with little regard for injury. Organizations like Little League stepped in and set up rules for the number of pitches and games young athletes could pitch, thus requiring teams to develop more pitchers. These rules had positive results, but two relatively recent events now threaten young pitchers: the advent of inexpensive radar guns and showcases (events for youth pitchers to demonstrate their throwing skill and velocity to college coaches and professional scouts). Formerly, radar guns were expensive and only owned by college coaches and professional baseball scouts. But radar guns have now become inexpensive and are heavily used. Young athletes throw for velocity with little regard for form. Youth coaches bring out their radar guns and test their athletes. Children look on the Internet to learn high-speed drills. To add to the problem, organizations (for profit) conduct Showcases. Showcases are held throughout the year but especially during the off-season when facilities are available, effectively creating year-round training for pitchers who play a seasonal sport. Further, scores are posted, increasing the influence of these Showcases.

Youth sport should be enjoyable and help prepare youngsters to play sport for a lifetime, but some sports may result in long-term problems. Sports medicine professionals encourage participants in sport to develop symmetry, to not overdevelop one part of the body while other parts are overlooked. Think of a sport like swimming; the swimmer has to develop both arms and legs equally, otherwise they would not swim in a straight line. Compare this with a sport like golf, in which an individual turns their body only counterclockwise (for the right-handed golfer), thousands of times. Now think of the young athlete who only plays golf; certainly they will develop asymmetry. Many youth sports are not asymmetrical, and sports like tennis, baseball, and softball pitching may result in future problems.

Burnout may not be a sport injury, but it results in the same thing: cessation of activity. Burnout has been defined to occur as a result of chronic stress that causes a young athlete to cease participation in a previously enjoyable activity. Specialization has been repeatedly cited as one factor that leads to burnout. One study found that children who grow up in the northern United States are more likely to become major league baseball players than kids from the South because they can't play baseball all year. Findings of the American Medical Society for Sports Medicine reported that children who specialize were found to be the first to quit their sport and ended up having higher inactivity rates as adults. There are multiple reasons for quitting, such as they aren't able to make the team, other interests prevail, athlete-sport mismatch, or it is just not fun and rewarding anymore and they are tired of focusing on one activity. There is no clear evidence that specialization results in superior athletic performance, but it does result in more injuries and burnout.

8. What tissues of the body can be affected by a sport injury?

The most common sport injuries occur to the soft tissues of the body. Muscles, tendons, and ligaments make up most of the soft tissue. Some joints also have sophisticated joint capsules that are lined with a membrane that secretes synovial fluid, a fluid that helps reduce joint friction by providing lubrication. Movable joints in the body are called synovial joints, and the ends of bones are all covered by a joint (hyaline) cartilage that protects bone ends and reduces friction. Some joints such as the shoulder and hip also have a labrum, a cartilaginous material that provides additional support for the head of the humerus and femur. Another injury site is the bone that can be acutely broken or suffer a stress fracture.

Muscles cause movement and are capable of infinite control from the tiniest tension, such as a small facial movement to maximum contraction of many muscles to lift heavy weights. Muscles come in all shapes and sizes dependent on their function. Long, slender muscles are responsible for long-range movement, while many small muscles are shaped to primarily provide stabilization. Regardless of shape or function, any muscle in the body can be injured, ranging from small tears to complete ruptures.

Each muscle is stimulated by a motor nerve to contract; when stimulated, the muscle tends to shorten. Muscles seldom work alone, as most movements of the body require multiple muscles. When we observe a high-velocity activity like sprinting, throwing, or kicking, it is little wonder that muscles get injured, as the contraction and relaxation of multiple muscles in a very short amount of time requires almost perfect synchronization. Another complicating factor is whether a muscle is uni- or biarticular. A uniarticular muscle only crosses one joint, while a biarticular muscle crosses two joints; biarticular muscles affect both joints they cross and tend to get injured more frequently.

Tendons are tough fibrous tissue that have elastic properties and connect each muscle to bone. When a muscle is stimulated, it tries to shorten, placing a pull on the tendon and subsequently to the bone to which it is attached. Tendons have elastic properties that allow it to briefly stretch before it begins to pull on the bone. When a muscle is quickly stretched, the tendon stretches and stores energy that is used for the following contraction. This is commonly called the stretch-shortening cycle (SSC), and athletes naturally use this to increase performance. Observe someone trying to jump as high as possible from a standing position. The first movement is a quick downward movement, flexing at the hip, knee, and ankle and stretching the quadriceps and Achilles tendon. The following muscle contraction is aided by the elastic energy stored in the tendon. Unfortunately, this huge increase in tension may tear or rupture the Achilles tendon.

Ligaments are dense bands of connective tissue that connect one bone to another. Injuries to ligaments are the most common musculoskeletal injury and routinely occur in knees, ankles, shoulders, and wrists. When a ligament is stretched too far, it can be torn just like muscles or tendons, leading to disruptions in joint mobility and stability. Ligaments primarily provide stabilization of joints by limiting joint movement at rest and during activity. Ligaments were once thought to be inactive, but they are not passive and respond to stress.

When a ligament is torn, it goes through an immediate healing process, but the process is relatively slow because of low blood supply. Ligaments can heal themselves, but one ligament that tends not to heal itself is the anterior cruciate ligament (ACL). The ACL forms an X with the posterior cruciate ligament (PCL), both attaching to the top of the tibia and the bottom of the femur, providing anterior and posterior stability. Unfortunately, when the ACL is ruptured, it is normally surgically repaired by replacing the ACL with other body tissues. Interestingly, there are many stories of individuals who have ruptured their ACLs and never had them repaired. These individuals seem to be able to cope with this injury without undue disability. However, these individuals do not normally return to the intense activity that caused the injury.

Bones are part of the musculoskeletal system, but they are the most resilient tissue and, under normal circumstances, are highly resistant to injury. Sport is a common cause of a broken bone, especially in those sports that involve contact. Football, ice hockey, and rugby are common sports that result in falling and collisions that break bones. It is important to understand that bone tissue is continuously changing, being broken down and renewing in a cycle that maintains bone strength. When this cycle is overwhelmed, the balance between break down and renewal is upset; a stress fracture is the result.

9. What are the basic stages of injury and healing, and how long do they last?

When an injury occurs, the body reacts within minutes to begin healing. The healing process involves four stages, each lasting anywhere from hours to months. Question 26 provides information on how each stage can be facilitated. When tissue is damaged, new tissue must form to replace it. Healing of muscle and tendon is not complete, and a collagen-based scar is normally formed. Skin and bone heal with the same type of tissue, and scar formation (if any) is limited. A fractured bone is often placed in a cast for three to eight weeks, and healing time depends on age, site of fracture, and type of fracture. Casting usually results in significant atrophy of the muscles involved. Remodeling of the bone will continue after the cast is removed. Table 3 indicates the basic stages in injury repair. The time frame depends on the type of injury and severity. A mild hamstring pull may take a week or so to heal, while a severe pull may take six months to repair. A ligament injury may take as long as a year, while injuries to nerves can take anywhere from a few days to many months. Nerve injuries that are far from the spine (such as the foot) take longer.

Table 3 The Four Stages of Healing

Phase	Major Activity	Duration
Bleeding	Stabilization of hemorrhage	Hours
Inflammatory phase	Cell migration to injury site to clear debris and begin repair.	1–7 days
Proliferative—repair and remodel	Development of collagenous scar and new vessels to repair and regenerate	1–3 weeks
Maturation	Organization and strengthening of new tissue and scar	3 weeks to a year

Bleeding will start immediately when a muscle is torn. Bleeding at the injury site results in swelling and pain. Range of motion of the joint is reduced because of the pressure. Occasionally, an athlete is injured during a competition but wishes to continue playing. The athlete is highly motivated to continue; the body experiences some analgesic effect, and the athlete is warm. Dependent on the severity, athletes frequently return to play, but activity at this point will stimulate more bleeding since blood flow to exercising areas is increased. Recovery time will be longer. As discussed in Question 26, RICE (rest, ice, compression, elevation) is the acronym for treatment during the bleeding period.

The acute inflammatory phase begins very quickly as multiple cells travel to the injured site to remove injured tissue. The usual signs of inflammation are redness, warmth, swelling, pain, and loss of function. These symptoms will diminish as this phase continues. Standard treatment for many years has been the use of anti-inflammatory medicines (NSAIDs) such as aspirin and ibuprofen, but recent work has suggested that thwarting the inflammatory phase is not the best practice. Tylenol (acetaminophen) may be a good substitute for pain relief, since it is not anti-inflammatory.

The proliferative stage begins about four to five days after the injury, and the injured tissue is cleared. During this stage, new collagen begins to form, and new blood vessels occur to help replenish the site. Meanwhile, it takes several weeks before the new structure begins to mature. Athletes can often begin to exercise during this stage, but this is a delicate period, as a reinjury starts the entire process over again, but it will take considerably longer time.

Finally, the maturation phase begins, which may take substantial time. When new collagen begins to form, it is very disorganized, and it takes time for it to become organized and for strength to return. Not only do the tissues need to regain their strength, but the injured muscle must also regain the proprioception (nervous control) that is necessary to regain form. Because of the complexity of muscle recruitment, the maturation phase requires appropriate rehabilitation techniques before the individual can return to full form.

Physicians diagnose muscle injuries and often classify sport injuries using a grading system. A physical exam is usually made, and the history of the injury is determined. There is usually swelling and bruising, and in some cases, the physician may feel a defect where the muscle is completely torn. Muscle injury almost always results in loss of strength and range of motion. Classification helps the staff assess the seriousness of the injury, and it may give some idea of the healing timeline. Most muscle injuries can be categorized into the following three grades:

Grade 1: The least serious involves only about 5 percent less of muscle fibers. There is mild loss of strength and motion, and these injuries take around two to three weeks to show considerable improvement.
Grade 2: This involves many more fibers, but the muscle is not ruptured; there is significant loss of strength and motion. Grade 2 injuries require two to three months to heal before a complete return to sport.
Grade 3: The most serious involves a complete rupture of muscle or tendon. Surgery is normally required to reattach the damaged muscle and tendon. Rehabilitation is long and arduous and takes about one year.

X-rays are often taken in cases of serious muscle strains even though muscles and tendons are not visible on an x-ray. Sometimes when a tendon or muscle is torn, a piece of the bone to which it is attached can also be pulled off. This is seen more frequently in young athletes, since the bones are not as developed. Other scanning techniques such as MRI are often used to establish the grade of injury.

10. What is the difference between an acute injury and an overuse injury?

Acute injuries are those injuries we normally observe when watching sports, the result of a single traumatic event. An athlete goes down, grabs his or her leg or shoulder, and is in obvious discomfort. The majority of acute injuries occur to the soft tissues of the musculoskeletal system and involve sprains and strains to the ankle, knee, and hip. The most

common acute injuries are sprained ankles, hamstring strains, knee ligament sprains, hip flexor strains, groin strains, and patella tendon pulls.
Although most acute injuries happen to the lower body, athletes also
suffer shoulder dislocations, broken and sprained wrists, broken collar-
bones, and concussions. As outlined in Question 9, bleeding and subsequent healing begins immediately and goes through the four outlined
phases. Acute injuries are normally graded from 1 to 3, with grade 3 being
the most serious. Acute injuries can also be catastrophic, defined by the
American Medical Association as a severe injury to the spine, spinal cord,
or brain. Football, cheerleading, and ice hockey are the three sports that
produce the most common catastrophic injuries. Catastrophic injuries are
based on three outcomes:

- Fatality
- Those causing permanent, severe functional disability
- Those causing severe head or neck trauma with no permanent
  disability

Overuse injuries are subtler and tend to creep up on the athlete. Athletes
often tend to overlook these slow starting injuries, but overuse injuries
can become chronic, leading to a long recovery time. When a person
starts training, stress is applied to the body. The body adapts by thick-
ening and strengthening the specific parts of the body that are involved;
muscles, tendons, ligaments, and bones get stronger. But when exercise is
applied in such a way that adaptation cannot occur and when the exercise
is excessive, recovery does not occur; maladaptation is the result. Overuse
injuries are normally caused by numerous, repeated, submaximal contractions, with insufficient rest to allow the specific tissue to recover.

By far most overuse injuries involve the tendon as well as the muscle/
tendon structure, but overuse injuries also occur in the covering of bone
(periosteum), such as shin splints, the bursa (bursitis), nerve (mechano-
sensitivity), and bone (stress fractures). Tendons can suffer acute injury
as well as overuse injury. An acute injury is caused by a sudden injury to
the tendon, usually a short-term injury involving inflammation and the
typical redness, warmth, and discomfort. "Tendinosis" is the term for an
overused tendon. Tendinosis does not involve inflammation and is more
structurally involved and longer lasting. The different terminology is in
the suffix, with "-itis" meaning inflammation, while "-osis" means dis-
eased or abnormal.

The first sign of overuse may be stiffness when you wake up in the
morning. This often goes away with a warm-up, but if exercise continues

without treatment, other signs begin to show. As discussed earlier, overuse injuries are subtle, and stiff tendons and muscles in the morning should not be overlooked if these symptoms continue (see Question 27 for treatment). Overuse injuries often develop in four stages.

1. Discomfort disappears during warm-up.
2. Discomfort may disappear during warm-up but reappears later during exercise.
3. Discomfort gets worse as exercise continues.
4. Discomfort is there all the time.

There is little question that the primary cause of overuse injuries involves training errors. Question 39 discusses how to avoid overuse injuries while continuing to train. Faulty technique is a common cause, as well as biomechanical misalignment, muscle imbalances, and incorrect equipment. Occasionally, athletes are not strong enough to participate in some strenuous training activities, and soft tissues are placed under too much stress.

All tendons can develop tendinosis, but the Achilles tendon is particularly susceptible because of the huge stress placed upon the tendon when running and jumping. Soccer players are particularly vulnerable. Jumping and landing also places specific stress on the patella tendon; throwing places substantial stress on the shoulder, elbow, and wrist. Tendons experience tiny tears in structure either at the place of insertion on the bone (insertional tendinosis) or in the middle of the tendon.

---◆❖◆---

Common Sport Injuries

11. What is a muscle strain, and which muscles are most likely to be strained?

How do you know you have strained a muscle (also called a pulled muscle or a muscle tear)? Muscle strains are rapid onset injuries; you immediately know something is wrong. If you simply wake up in the morning and have muscle pain, it's not a muscle strain. A muscle cramp is not a muscle strain. Muscles can also be bruised, but a bruise is not a strain. Muscle pulls most frequently occur where the muscle and tendon meet. The following checklist may help you determine if you have a strained muscle:

- Did the pain occur immediately—did you have an "oh no" moment?
- Is there pain at a specific point in the muscle?
- Is there swelling? Injured fibers will quickly swell.
- Is it flushed and hot?
- Is there deformation?

All these symptoms do not have to occur, but the first symptom is the best predictor.

What muscles are most often strained? Certainly, strains of the hamstrings are the most common and often the most troublesome. First, so many sport activities require running, and it is difficult to run with a torn hamstring. Second, hamstring strains tend to recur, one sign that the muscle tear was never really healed. Muscles that cross two joints, biarticular, are more susceptible, as their actions are more complex. Also, it's the bigger muscles that are normally torn. The following list indicates the most frequently torn muscles:

- Hamstrings (the three muscles in the back of the thigh)
- Rectus femoris (the most superficial of the quadriceps group—the only biarticular muscle of the quads)
- Gastrocnemius (calf muscle—attaches the heel to the back of the knee)
- Lumbar paraspinals (thick columns of muscle on each side of the lumbar spine)
- Biceps

Regarding recovery from a muscle tear, the more fibers torn, the more the serious it is. Complete rupture of a muscle is rare. Question 9 presented the stages of healing as well as how to grade an injury. Grade 1 recovery time is about three to six weeks. Grade 2 strains may take several months, while Grade 3 is even longer and normally requires surgery. In most cases, a scar is left, one reason the muscle may tear again.

Muscle injuries occur frequently in all sports and at all levels of sport. In the past few decades, year-round training in sport has increased, and it is not surprising that this has taken a toll on muscles as well. How much training a muscle can take without injury is unknown. What is known is that muscles cannot be in top condition all year; a period of rest must follow intense bouts or seasons of vigorous activity. To understand muscle injury, one must understand the different ways muscle can contract. Muscles have the ability to completely relax, no tension, but when stimulated by a motor nerve, they can undergo three types of contraction: static, concentric, or eccentric. Most muscle strains occur during an eccentric contraction.

When a muscle is stimulated, it tends to shorten. Oftentimes a muscle contracts but does not move. This is called a static (isometric) contraction. A number of exercises exist that require static contraction. For example, side planks are isometric exercises. Many yoga poses are static, which involve muscles contracting statically to maintain the required position.

Typically the muscle contracts, overcomes resistance, and shortens. A muscle contraction that results in muscle shortening is called a concentric contraction. But there are times when the muscle creates tension but lengthens; this is called an eccentric contraction. Most weight room exercises have a concentric-eccentric sequence. A simple example of this is when you do an arm curl. Let's say you pick up a dumbbell to do an arm curl. You contract your biceps; the muscle shortens, and the elbow flexes and moves upward. Now you want to lower the weight; gravity is pulling it down, but you don't want to just drop it, so you reduce the tension in the biceps and the weight lowers. The fibers in the biceps get longer under tension—an eccentric contraction of the biceps.

Muscle injury does not normally occur during this simple concentric-eccentric sequence, but it happens when a muscle is attempting to slow down a high-speed movement or when a muscle is attempting to absorb a force. Observe an individual landing from a jump; the hip, knee, and ankle all flex over a distance, slowly absorbing the stopping force. The muscles that cause knee extension (the quadriceps) contract eccentrically to absorb the stopping force. Likewise, the Achilles tendon and calf muscle lengthen to absorb the shock of landing—a common way the Achilles tendon and calf muscle are torn. Another example, and the one that causes a torn hamstring, is when an individual is sprinting. During sprinting, the back leg moves forward quickly, and the knee rapidly extends. In order to protect the knee joint, the muscle that causes knee flexion, the hamstring group, contracts eccentrically, slowing down the rapid knee extension. This is when the hamstring tears. Observing someone running at top speed, one has to marvel at the complex timing required to contract and relax the muscles in the front and back of the leg. There is little surprise that occasionally this sequence gets out of synchronization, causing undue tension in the hamstring; the result is a torn hamstring. Individuals who are not familiar with sprinting tear their hamstrings easily. Fatigue and a lack of warm-up are common reasons for a torn hamstring. Fatigue is the enemy of neurological control.

12. What is a sprain, and which ligaments are most commonly sprained?

The most common musculoskeletal injury is a sprain, an injury to the ligament (or ligaments) that crosses a joint to connect one bone to another. As indicated in Question 8, ligaments are dense bands of connective tissue that stabilize joints and guide joint movement. A sprain is an acute injury, when an individual feels an immediate disruption in a joint. Pain and swelling happen almost immediately followed by a limited ability to move the injured joint. Occasionally, the individual may hear or feel a "pop" at the time of injury. Normally, this involves a more serious sprain and a possible rupture of the ligament.

The evidence is very clear that ankle sprains are the most common sport injury, often caused by walking or running on an uneven surface or landing awkwardly on one foot. Sports that involve a lot of jumping (and landing), such as volleyball, basketball, and soccer, are especially problematic. The common ankle sprain is on the outside (lateral) side of the foot, often involving more than one ligament. We often see athletic trainers or physicians examining a knee and palpating the ankle for injury sites. The purpose of this examination is to determine which ligaments are damaged, as some ligaments take longer to heal. Sportscasters frequently talk about an athlete having a high ankle sprain as being problematic. When an athlete sprains the ligament that connects the bottom of the tibia to the bottom of the fibula, this is a high ankle sprain; it takes longer to heal.

There are four major ligaments in the knee: one ligament on each side of the knee and two cruciate ligaments that are inside the knee connecting the tibia to the femur. The broad ligament on the inside of the knee (medial collateral ligament [MCL]) is the most commonly sprained knee ligament. This ligament is often injured by receiving a blow to the outside of the knee, stretching the MCL beyond normal range. The MCL is also injured when the lower leg is planted and the body twists in the opposite direction. Fortunately, the MCL is very good at healing itself. An injury to the anterior cruciate ligament (ACL) is the second-most common knee sprain. As discussed in Question 8, injuries to the ACL are problematic, often requiring surgery and a long rehabilitation. The ACL is most often injured during deceleration, such as when stopping, turning, or landing. Most ACL injuries are noncontact and frequently occur in sports like soccer, basketball, football, and lacrosse.

Also frequently injured is the wrist, caused by landing on an outstretched arm when falling. The thumb is another common sprain area for downhill skiers and tennis players. A sprain that occurs in the shoulder is mistakenly called a separated shoulder. This is a sprain of the ligament that connects the collarbone (clavicle) to the shoulder blade (scapula). This injury occurs when falling on the point of the shoulder, common in football. Like all ligament injuries, a separated shoulder ranges from mild to a complete rupture of the ligament.

The treatment for a sprain is discussed in Question 26. It usually takes 5–14 days to recover from a grade 1 sprain and 4–6 weeks for a grade 2 sprain. Most sprains do not require surgery, but grade 3 strains may require reattachment by surgery. Unfortunately, some ankle sprains may take as long as a year or two to heal, and some present lifetime instability. Injured athletes often ask if they should continue to walk when recovering from a sprained knee or ankle. The answer depends somewhat on the degree of damage, but one should restrict movement during the early stages to reduce swelling. But following this early stage, some exercise is recommended, since exercise promotes blood flow and removal of dead tissue and swelling. The exercise may help with stiffness but should not cause more damage. Pain is a symptom of damage.

13. What are tendonitis and tendinosis?

Question 8 describes tendons as the tissue that connects muscles to bones. Tendons are tough fibers that also have elastic properties. Since tendons transmit the force of muscle contractions to bones, the integrity of tendons is of paramount importance for athletes and anyone engaging in exercise. Like many tissues, tendons can adapt to exercise stress, but tendons can maladapt as a result of excessive load, incurring an acute or overuse injury. Load is the key to injury, but load can come in more than one form. For instance, an abrupt increase in training volume is the most common form of increased load, but another tendon problem relates to form. Individuals who play a sport with improper biomechanics often place excess load on one body part, a part that tends to maladapt. This is often the case for novice tennis players who place disproportionate stress on their elbows and shoulders. Some baseball pitchers try to throw at high velocities without good form, hurting their elbows and shoulders. In addition, when recovering from an injury, athletes might change their biomechanical form, placing more stress on other soft tissues.

"Tendonitis" is the most common word used when referring to tendon injuries. However, most tendon injuries are probably not tendonitis (an acute injury) but tendinosis (an overuse injury). All tendon injuries are tendinopathies, referring to a range of tendon injuries, going from a short-term inflammatory phase to a long-term phase that may result in tissue death or rupture.

Tendonitis refers to tendon problems related to inflammation; the suffix, "itis," means inflammation, a condition that stimulates the inflammatory response. Tendonitis occurs most often when there is an abrupt increase in load. Let's say a competitive badminton player has taken a month off and then goes out and plays three long singles games. The tendons in the elbow and shoulder might easily inflame as a response. A jogger decides to add sprints up a steep hill to improve fitness; the response might be an inflamed Achilles tendon. Tendonitis is more an acute injury, but it is not a sudden-onset injury like a hamstring tear. Tendonitis is a bit subtler, creeping up on you the next day or two.

Tendinosis is also a tendinopathy, but it's different from tendonitis, primarily with regard to time. It takes time to develop tendinosis. When a tendon is repeatedly stressed without appropriate rest, the tendon maladapts, resulting in a weaker, disorganized tendon. Inflammation is not the problem, but a degeneration of the tendon's fibers is. Conditions like tennis elbow or runner's knee are mostly tendinosis.

Recovery time for tendinopathies is somewhat dependent on when the condition was recognized and treated. Athletes need to be aware of the difference between tendon pain and muscle soreness. Tenderness to the tendon upon palpation, pain when exercising, weakness, and mild swelling are symptoms that the tendon has experienced excess load. If the individual ignores the symptoms, healing takes longer time. Recovery time for tendonitis can be just several days to 6 weeks, while healing in tendinosis can be as brief as 6–10 weeks if treatment is started immediately. Recovery from tendinopathies can take months if the participant ignores symptoms and keeps on doing the activity that caused the initial problem.

14. What is a fracture, and which bones are most likely to be fractured?

When we think of bone injury, a broken bone normally comes to mind. Fractures are defined as a loss of continuity of a bone and may be a complete or incomplete break. The human body has 206 bones, and falling, collisions, and sport may break any of them. Contact sports such as football, ice hockey, and rugby result in the most broken bones. Bone fractures are also common in downhill skiing. The collarbone (clavicle) is the most commonly broken bone, primarily because of its location as the contact bone between the upper arm and the ribs. The collarbone is frequently broken when falling, as the individual attempts to break the fall by putting their hand out. Broken arms are the second-most common fracture and may result in multiple fractures in one bone. The ankle and foot are also common fracture sites. Since the foot contains 25 percent of all the bones in the body, fractures in the foot are not unusual. Broken ankles are the most common fracture in the foot.

Falling is the normal cause of fracture in the upper or lower bones in the arm or in the wrist. Often, breaks in the wrist involve multiple bones (carpals). Falling occurs not only in many contact sports but also in activities like skateboarding, downhill skiing, and cycling. Individuals who play other sports that result in falling should practice falling in such a way to reduce the impact on just one part of the body. Learn to fall by rolling and absorbing the force over a greater distance and body parts.

While all athletes (and especially dancers) are susceptible to avulsion fractures, children are more at risk. Avulsion fractures occur when a part of the bone is actually torn from the primary bone. These often occur in tuberosities or tubercles, small bumps on the bones that develop during growth as ligaments and muscles pull on the bone. Since it is during growth when these bony structures develop, children are susceptible. Occasionally avulsion fractures are misdiagnosed as a torn muscle, so an x-ray should be obtained.

In Question 4, injuries to the growth plate (epiphysis) were discussed. The growth plate is at the end of the bone and is two to five times weaker than other parts of the bone. Only preadolescents and adolescents are at risk of epiphyseal injuries, and 15–30 percent of all bone injuries in children occur in the epiphysis. Prognosis for epiphyseal injuries is good, but treatment must start immediately and usually involves immobilization by casting. Improper treatment can result in lifelong problems, such as unequal growth and bones more susceptible to injury.

The immediate symptoms of fractures are pain and swelling. Some fractures are very painful. Applying ice at this time is recommended. Immobilization by a cast normally follows, but some fractures require realignment. This is normally a surgical procedure and can involve more complicated treatment, such as the insertion of rods, plates, or screws to hold the bones in place while healing. The Cleveland Clinic suggests that the average time for a bone to heal is six to eight weeks, but this depends on several factors; fracture severity is the most important. During immobilization, significant atrophy (muscle wasting) occurs, so rehabilitation involves exercise that supports the maturation phase of bone healing as well as muscle strengthening. Continuing to exercise during immobilization is recommended, plus a healthy diet including the recommended calcium intake (1,300 mg/day for teenagers and 1,000 mg/day for young adults). Smoking compromises bone health.

15. What are stress fractures, and who tends to get them?

Bone is very adaptable to stress; regular exercise results in bones that are stronger and more resistant to injury, but bone can maladapt as well. Bone is in a continuous state of change, constantly being broken down and renewed. Normally, the breakdown-synthesis process is in equilibrium, but maladaptation occurs when the equilibrium between breakdown and synthesis is out of balance, when breakdown overwhelms synthesis. In such a condition, the bone begins to fail, and if not corrected, a stress fracture results. A stress fracture is an overuse injury, as the bone is susceptible when the stress of the mechanical load is very high and rest is insufficient for synthesis. Stress fractures make up about 2 percent of all sport injuries.

Errors in training are the principal cause of stress fractures. The most common error is a rapid increase in training volume. Excess fatigue also tires muscle, causing an increase in bone stress. Stress fractures typically occur in high-impact, repetitive activity sports, such as running, basketball, and track. A typical stress fracture is often related to an increase in activity, particularly at the beginning of the season. A new season begins, athletes and coaches are enthusiastic, motivation is high, and athletes are less trained and tend to overdo it. Another example is when an athlete transfers from one sport to another. For example, athletes on swim teams are very fit and have excellent cardiovascular endurance, but they may have been training in an environment that places little stress on bones in the lower leg. Swim season ends, and the swimmer goes out for track and overdoes the training; bones in the foot and lower leg begin to fail. Changes in surface without a concomitant reduction in volume are a frequent problem. In addition, improper footwear, bunions, blisters, or tendonitis may change how one runs, placing extra stress on bones.

Like most overuse injuries, stress fracture symptoms are rather subtle at the beginning. You hardly notice it, but it tends to worsen with time. There is specific tenderness at the point of injury and occasionally mild swelling. In the beginning, pain resolves when at rest, but when pain becomes more persistent, it is time to get evaluated. X-rays do not really show a stress fracture but may show some disturbance; bone or MRI scans are typically used to diagnose a stress fracture.

Most stress fractures occur to the foot, lower leg, and hip. The foot is particularly problematic. But stress fractures in the upper body also occur, especially in activities such as high-speed throwing (pitching), gymnastics, and rowing. Most stress fractures will heal on their own if one simply stops doing the activity that caused it, but this is problematic when the stress fracture is in the foot, as the individual needs to remain mobile. In such situations, the injured person needs to wear very supportive shoes or even a walking boot. Athletes are not going to work their way out of a stress fracture as the fracture will not heal without rest. Generally, it takes about four to six weeks to heal most bones, but some bones take longer. Resuming activity is somewhat tricky, as you do not want to reinjure the same bone, resulting in an even lengthier recovery. Prognosis is good if the athlete is careful and follows the treatment plan.

Females get more stress fractures than men, especially if accompanied by an eating disorder. Studies on military recruits show that women recruits are as much as 10 times more likely to receive a stress fracture. Much of the difference is explained by body weight and fitness. Studies comparing male and female athletes are not nearly so dramatic. In fact, women who are fit have normal weight and bone health and who have a regular menstrual cycle are at relatively low risk of stress fracture.

Menstrual regularity is particularly important for the overall health of female athletes as well as bone health. Hormonal balance is an important component of the equilibrium between breakdown and resynthesis; bone development needs hormonal balance. Women who have lost menstrual regularity are at high risk of a stress fracture as well as long-term bone health. Females have a narrow window in which to develop bone; when a regular cycle is lost because of excess exercise, females lose part of that window and may reach maturity with bones that are less dense than normal. Menstrual irregularity is related to intense exercise as well as a poor diet, stress, and the overall energy drain of exercise and daily requirements.

16. What is a concussion, how do you get one, and what are the risks associated with an undiagnosed concussion?

A concussion is a traumatic brain injury (TBI) caused by a blow or hit to the body or head that causes the head and brain to move rapidly back and forth. A sudden movement may cause the brain to bounce or twist in the skull, stretching or damaging brain cells. Common causes are severe blows to the head, such as those occurring in football, ice hockey, and soccer, or a fall in which the skull strikes the ground and the brain moves within the skull. Concussion is not uncommon, affecting about 128 people per 100,000 in the United States per year. Concussions are normally labeled as "mild brain injuries" because a single concussion is not life-threatening.

Two conditions can change a mild brain injury to something more permanent. As discussed in Question 4, multiple concussions over the years can take a huge toll on the brain. Chronic traumatic encephalopathy (CTE) is a degenerative brain disease that is related to repeated concussions. CTE is very serious, causing serious dementia, depression, and memory loss. CTE takes about 15 years to develop. Secondary impact syndrome (SIS) is a second condition that may turn a mild brain injury to one much more serious. SIS occurs when an individual receives a second concussion while still experiencing postconcussive symptoms from an initial concussion. SIS is relatively rare but can cause serious problems such as serious bleeding in the brain, swelling, and even death.

Diagnosis (covered in Question 28) is critical regarding the safe treatment of concussions. The recent publicity of suicides by famous athletes suffering from CTE has improved the awareness of blows to the head. Athletic teams in schools have concussion protocols in place, improving diagnosis. Unfortunately, recent studies have found very limited knowledge of concussion symptoms. One study found that more than 50 percent of high school athletes and 70 percent of collegiate athletes did not report concussions sustained during football. The athletes were not aware of the symptoms. Many people receive concussions in nonschool sports where there is no supervision by an athletic trainer or physician.

Men's football and women's soccer clearly result in the greatest number of concussions. While the rate of concussions may be higher in other sports, many more athletes play football and soccer. Men's rugby and women's ice hockey have a higher incidence of concussion but fewer participants. The incidence of concussion is much higher in games than practice, but one approach to reducing concussions is to reduce contact during practice. An effective procedure to reduce concussions is a reduction of contact in practice.

Restricting contact in high school and college athletics has reduced the number of concussions during practice. However, most of these restrictions are only practiced during the competitive season. Such restrictions are normally not followed during off-season or spring training. Youth football is another concern, as youth football associations are often not well organized with vague rules about physical contact. Further, coaches of youth teams are often volunteers with no real coaching credentials.

Concussions remain a mild brain injury, as there is little evidence that a single concussion has any long-term effect. The recovery from a single concussion is satisfactory as long as the injured party follows the recommended treatment (Question 28). Multiple concussions over many years may present very serious long-lasting problems that negatively affect one's quality of life.

17. What is the rotator cuff, and what happens when you injure it?

The shoulder is called a ball-and-socket joint, as the head of the humerus (upper arm) fits into a socket on the upper end of the scapula (shoulder blade). Unlike the hip, another ball-and-socket joint, the shoulder socket is quite shallow, allowing humans extensive shoulder mobility. This mobility comes with a risk: the absence of a deep socket and bony structure to stabilize the shoulder. The shoulder relies on soft tissues like ligaments, tendons, and muscles for stability.

Four relatively small muscles come off the front or rear surface of the scapula to attach to the head of the humerus: the rotator cuff muscles. Although the rotator cuff muscles do aid to rotate the humerus, a significant action of each muscle is to hold the humerus in the socket, to stabilize. The rotator cuff muscles are as follows:

- Supraspinatus—is at the top of the shoulder and helps raise the arm
- Infraspinatus—is in the back of the shoulder and helps rotate outward
- Teres minor—is the smallest rotator cuff and assists the infraspinatus
- Subscapularis—is in the front of the shoulder and helps rotate inward

Like any muscle or tendon, a rotator cuff muscle or its tendon can be torn. Tears of the rotator cuff muscles are the most common of the shoulder injuries and can be the result of an acute injury or an overuse injury. Most rotator cuff injuries are related to athletes who perform extensively overhead; baseball pitchers and tennis players are particularly susceptible. However, any athlete can receive an acute rotator cuff injury by falling or lifting a heavy weight overhead. As individuals age, the incidence of rotator cuff injury increases significantly.

In addition to a muscle tear, three other rotator cuff problems are fairly common:

- Tendinosis (or tendonitis): described in Question 13.
- Bursitis: there are small sacs of fluid that surround the rotator cuff and tendon. When faced with excessive repetition and little rest, these sacs become irritated and inflamed.
- Impingement: a common overuse shoulder ailment and can involve both tendonitis and bursitis. As the muscles repeatedly contract, the tendon and muscle swells, rubbing against the top of the scapula and the bursa. Swimmers are particularly susceptible. Physical therapy is the primary treatment along with injections of steroid to reduce inflammation. The outcome is promising, but impingement that does not respond to therapy may need surgery.

An injury to one or more of the rotator cuff muscles seriously compromises shoulder performance. While there are other big shoulder muscles, the rotator cuff muscles are important aids. As discussed in Question 8, muscles seldom work alone, and all shoulder movements involve the rotator cuff. The fluid motion that is apparent in activities like throwing, hitting overhead, or swimming is not replicated when the rotator cuff is injured.

Early symptoms include the following:

- Tending to avoid certain activities because they cause pain
- Difficulty achieving full range of motion
- Difficulty sleeping on one shoulder
- Pain when reaching overhead
- Weakness
- Distress when reaching behind your back

Diagnosing rotator cuff injuries often involves a physician or physical therapist, putting one through a series of mobility tests, and attempting to determine specific weaknesses or reduced range of motion. Ultrasound and MRI imaging are also used.

Recovery from a rotator cuff tear obviously depends on the severity of the damage. Recovery usually takes about two to four weeks, but it can take months if there has been considerable overuse. Rest is often recommended. Occasionally, the athlete may wear a sling for a few days. Recovery requires specific exercises designed by a competent therapist.

A completely torn rotator cuff muscle or tendon will not heal on its own. Surgery is the standard treatment for a complete rupture. Recovery from surgery lasts four to six months during which time the individual must be patient, allowing the surgery to heal, for the tendons to reattach. Normally the individual must wear a sling attached to the trunk for about five weeks. Extensive and systematic rehabilitation by a specialist is the key to recovery.

18. What other injuries can affect the shoulder?

As discussed in Question 17, the shoulder is capable of extensive mobility, but it is also unstable, relying heavily on ligaments, tendons, and muscles to stabilize this important joint. Technically, the shoulder is composed of the humerus (upper arm), the scapula (shoulder blade), and the clavicle (collar bone). Injuries to any of these bones or the soft tissues supporting them are considered an injury to the shoulder. In Question 17, injury to the rotator cuff muscles was identified as the most common shoulder injury. However, other shoulder injuries also occur.

Broken Clavicle

A broken clavicle is quite common, and the clavicle is the most frequently broken bone in the body. The typical mechanism for such an injury is falling with an outstretched hand or on the point of the shoulder. When the hand hits the ground, the force travels through the arm, to the clavicle, and to the sternum (breastbone). The clavicle is the weak link and tends to break. Clavicle breaks are more common in young people, since the bone does not completely harden until around age 20.

The main symptom of a clavicular break is pain that increases when you move your arm, tenderness, and swelling, and sometimes a small bump appears. Most breaks to the collarbone heal well within six to eight weeks with ice, a sling, and rehabilitation. It then takes about the same time to fully return to preinjury status. A complicated break might require surgery.

Dislocated Shoulder

A dislocated shoulder occurs when the head of the humerus will pop out of the shoulder socket. When this happens, the shoulder needs to be reduced, put back in place by a medical professional. Anesthesia is normally not required, and relief is immediate. The shoulder is the most frequently dislocated joint in the body and occurs in contact sports as well as sports in which individuals may experience a hard fall, such as downhill skiing. Extreme rotation that might happen in kayaking or wrestling may result in a shoulder dislocation.

The primary symptom of a shoulder dislocation is substantial pain as well as deformity and an inability to move the arm. If a dislocation is suspected, one should put the arm in a sling and go to the emergency room or urgent care center. It is important to reduce the dislocation as soon as you can. Since a shoulder dislocation that is not reduced can cause nerve or blood flow problems, a dislocation in a wilderness area may present serious problems, one reason a member of the traveling party should have emergency medical training.

Following reduction, a sling is often utilized for a few days to allow the shoulder to rest, after which gentle range-of-motion exercises should begin. You should begin to resume normal activities within about two weeks, but it will take about 12–16 weeks to completely recover.

Subluxing Shoulder

You sublux your shoulder when the head of the humerus temporarily moves out of the socket but returns on its own. This is a fairly common shoulder injury, accounting for about 20 percent of shoulder injuries. A typical subluxation occurs when the head of the humerus moves forward (anterior subluxation) and then moves back into place. Unfortunately, neither conservative rehabilitation techniques nor surgery has been overwhelmingly effective in treating a subluxating shoulder. Athletes who experience repeated subluxations frequently change sports, as the fear of repeated subluxations overwhelms one's ability to enjoy the activity.

Labral Tears

These tears affect shoulder strength and range of motion. The labrum is a piece of rubbery fibrocartilage that helps hold the head of the humerus in place. Labral tears are often the result of fairly intense overhead work over time. The common labral tear is called a SLAP tear. SLAP is defined as follows:

- S: superior (above)
- L: labrum
- A: anterior (front)
- P: posterior (back)

SLAP tears are common among baseball and softball players, who do a lot of intense overhand throwing. People who do a lot of overhead weight training are also susceptible. SLAP tears are often associated with the biceps, since the long tendon of the biceps attaches to the shoulder at the labrum, and when the bicep tendon is torn, the labrum is pulled away. Labral tears respond reasonably well to physical therapy, but a severe SLAP tear will probably require surgery, taking 12–18 months to recover. Some never recover their preinjury form.

19. What are the most common causes of pain in the elbow?

The anatomy of the elbow is somewhat like the knee in that the long bone of the upper arm (humerus) articulates with the two smaller bones in the forearm: the ulna and the radius. The ulna is on the inside (medial), and the radius is on the outside (lateral). The elbow is a hinge joint and allows only flexion and extension, but just below the elbow, the radius can rotate around the ulna through pronation and supination. Pronation is when the hand is turned from palm up to palm down, and supination is the reverse. In many overhead movements of the upper arm, flexion and extension are accompanied by either pronation or supination; such movements are complicated.

Similar to the knee, there are collateral ligaments on each side of the elbow. Of these, the ulnar collateral ligament (UCL) is on the inside, connecting the humerus to the ulna, and is the ligament most often injured. The UCL undergoes extreme stress during overhand throwing, tennis serving, and volleyball spiking and serving. The ulnar nerve crosses behind the elbow and controls the muscles of the hand and feeling in the small and ring fingers. The ulnar nerve can be injured by falling or overuse.

Like any joint, soft tissues are responsible for a considerable amount of elbow stability and can be injured, resulting in pain and loss of function. Bones of the elbow can be broken. The most common elbow injuries include the following.

Broken Arm

A broken elbow is a misnomer, since a broken elbow is really a broken upper arm or a break of one of the two forearm bones. A direct blow can cause a break in any of these three bones, but falling is the common cause of a fracture. Many fractures of the forearm simply require a cast and sling, but some actually require realignment. Breaks of the upper arm do not normally require surgery, as the bones are not separated, but a sling is worn during healing.

The prognosis for broken arm bones is generally good if treated early. Complicated breaks may result in nerve damage, and stiffness is normally encountered, requiring physical therapy following removal of the cast or sling. Six to twelve weeks is the typical time required for a broken arm to heal.

Ulnar Collateral Ligament

The UCL is the predominant ligament on the inside of the elbow. As the arm comes vigorously forward during overhand actions such as throwing a baseball, the strain on the UCL is extensive. Injury to the UCL is primarily caused by excessive repetitions over long periods. Individuals who do not participate in overhand activities rarely injure the UCL The most common symptom of injury to the UCL is pain on the inside of the elbow when throwing, as well as a decrease in velocity.

For many years in baseball, pitchers who lost velocity were said to have a "dead arm." This condition was normally caused by a rupture in the

UCL, usually resulting in the end of a pitcher's career. In 1974, an orthopedic surgeon named Frank Jobe tried a new surgery on Tommy John, a baseball pitcher, replacing the ruptured UCL with a tendon from another part of the body. Jobe put the chances of success at 1–100 percent. Up until that point, John had been a successful pitcher, winning 124 games. Following the surgery, John won 164 games, retiring in 1989 at age 46. Tommy John surgery, as it is called today, is quite common with a success rate from 85 to 92 percent. Following surgery, about one year of rehabilitation is necessary for pitchers to return to action. Surprisingly, 57 percent of Tommy John surgeries are on 15- to 19-year-old boys, mostly caused by too much pitching, poor biomechanics, and too little time off. About 25 percent of major league baseball pitchers eventually have Tommy John surgery.

Golfer's Elbow

Also known as medial epicondylitis, it's caused by damage to the muscles and tendons that control your forearm and wrist. Pronation of the forearm is an important movement in sport. The muscles that cause pronation primarily originate on the epicondyle (bump on the inside of the elbow). They can become inflamed because of improper hitting (such as in golf), excessive hitting, excessive use of topspin in tennis, and an improper warm-up. Individuals who practice extensively without rest are particularly susceptible.

This is a fairly common injury but not really serious. Usually icing and rest allow the soft tissues to heal. Proper equipment is important along with warming up with softer shots before swinging a golf club at full speed. Golfers should take care not to hit the ball if the surface is questionable, such as a root or rock under the ball.

Tennis Elbow

Also known as lateral epicondylitis, tennis elbow is similar to golfer's elbow, but it's on the outside of the elbow. Tennis players are predisposed because of the stress placed on the outside of the elbow when hitting a backhand. Tennis elbow is an overuse injury caused by excessive repetition, but poor biomechanics are another cause. The backhand in tennis should involve the kinetic chain (Question 41) so that the force is generated through the body from the ground, thereby reducing the stress on the elbow. Tennis players who hit a backhand with excess elbow flexion at contact are very vulnerable to tennis elbow.

Primary symptoms include pain on the outside of the elbow when play-ing, pain when shaking hands or holding an object, and some swelling. If not treated early, tennis elbow can become serious with surgery as a last resort.

Ulnar Nerve Compression

The ulnar nerve runs at the back of the elbow and is vulnerable, espe-cially when falling. The spot where the nerve runs is often called the "funny bone"; at this point, the nerve is close to the surface. So athletes in football and rugby are susceptible, especially those athletes who fall and do not wear elbow padding. Learning to fall properly is a good way to avoid ulnar nerve compression. If there is frequent tingling in hands and fingers, as well as muscle wasting, a medical evaluation should be con-ducted. Ulnar nerve compression can become quite serious, even requir-ing surgery.

20. What are the most common problems with the back and trunk muscles?

The spine is one of the most important areas of the body, as the spine surrounds the spinal cord, sending and receiving neurological signals to and from the brain. Spinal pain can be one of the most debilitating problems for athletes. Small vertebrae stack on top of one another, each separated by a cartilaginous disc, to form the spinal column. The three areas of the spine include the cervical (top 7 vertebrae), thoracic (next 12 with attached ribs), and lumbar (bottom 5). The lumbar, lower back, is the most problematic. Problems with the thoracic spine are rare, as little movement occurs due to the attached ribs. The cervical area is at risk from falling, a whiplash effect from starting or stopping quickly, or a direct blow. The cervical vertebrae are also the most mobile and can suffer twisting stress.

In the back (posterior), multiple skeletal muscles (erector spinae) run up and down the spine and ribs. Low back pain (LBP) is often related to these muscles and tendons. In the front (anterior), the trunk is pri-marily stabilized by the five abdominal muscles: rectus abdominus in the middle and external and internal oblique muscles on each side. Verte-brae can withstand considerable vertical stress but not significant hor-izontal stress. Many sports can result in spinal problems, but especially those sports that produce considerable stress such as football, gymnastics, and rowing. Sports that involve numerous repetitions of twisting stress like golf and tennis may result in asymmetrical development resulting in back pain. Weight machines that require twisting horizontal stress can be problematic.

LBP is by far the most common spinal problem. It is usually caused by a variety of factors, including the sport in which one is engaged, posture, weak trunk muscles, and faulty biomechanical patterns. Treatment for LBP should be comprehensive and only done by well-trained personnel. Traumatic injuries to the lower back have been reduced because of the increased concern and rule changes to protect the head and spine, but sports that involve tackling still result in acute injuries to the lower back. Most low back injuries are related to overuse. LBP is often associated with a specific movement, such as rowing, specific weight training exercises, running, or cycling. Treatment involves the typical treatment for overuse injury. However, some athletes develop what is called insidious LBP, which is the result of other factors such as poor study posture, poor sleep, and stress, coupled with athletic activities. Insidious LBP must be treated by first discovering the nonathletic activity that causes problems. Typical therapy is not successful.

Sport accounts for about 10 percent of all injuries to the cervical spine, but about one-half of the entire population will have some form of neck pain in their lives. Sports that include the most cervical spine (neck) problems are football, rugby, diving, equestrian, and snow sports. Many cervical injuries are traumatic, involving a single event that ranges from an injury to soft tissue, fracture of the cervical vertebrae, to paralysis. Cervical injuries can also involve overuse such as when an individual must hold their neck in a fixed position for extensive periods such as in a winter sliding sport (luge, bobsled).

In the event of an injury to the neck, the first thing is to eliminate any serious problem that may result in more damage. In the case of injury to muscles and tendons, the first phase of treatment is to establish range of motion. This treatment normally starts immediately followed by exercises to strengthen neck muscles. Isometric (static) exercises are first used, followed by resistance activities that involve motion. The time period to return to play is varied and should require complete recovery of motion, strength, lack of pain, and form. LBP is normally treated like any other sprain or strain, beginning with rest and a return to exercise to help strengthen and improve range of motion. A common question about LBP is whether to increase bed rest; the answer is an unequivocal no by medical personnel. Individuals with LBP should continue to move as much as possible.

A fairly common injury mentioned during television commentary on football is a stinger. A stinger is a sport-related injury to nerves around the neck and shoulder, usually caused by a collision. Stinger symptoms include painful electrical sensations radiating through one of the arms. Although the stinger is usually a spine injury, it is never a spinal cord injury. Stingers tend to resolve rather quickly, but the athlete is more at risk of subsequent stingers that can lead to muscle weakness. A combination of ice and heat is often used during recovery along with a cervical collar to rest and support the neck.

Sport participation causes most back and spine injuries, but individuals involved in weightlifting and intense calisthenic programs are also at risk. As mentioned earlier, the spine is well suited to withstanding vertical stress, but a shear (horizontal) stress is not well tolerated. Excessive flexion in the lumbar spine can cause LBP as well as a herniated disk. Many fitness gyms have weight machines in which the user is supported. In such cases, injury is infrequent. But when individuals are using free weights, the possibility of injury increases, particularly true for exercises like the dead lift, squat, clean, and overhead press. Although these exercises are often labeled as being superior for sport performance, many athletes are not sufficiently skilled to prevent injury to the back. The primary problem is that the weight places excessive horizontal stress (torque) on the spine because the user flexes too much in the lumbar spine, one important reason professional instruction is important.

Some calisthenic exercises can also cause LBP, especially for those individuals who excessively perform abdominal exercises. The misplaced belief that highly defined abdominal muscles are synonymous with fitness has led many participants to leave the gym with LBP. Excessive sit-ups, leg raises, and trunk twisting crunches can result in injury to the lower back. A healthy back and spine is dependent on proper exercise, activities that are not excessive or asymmetrical and that improve or maintain flexibility and strength.

21. What are the most common problems with the hip and thigh?

The large muscles of the thighs, lower back, and buttocks support the pelvic girdle. Since these muscles are all relatively strong, it takes significant force to cause an acute injury. Injuries in this area are overuse and acute; strains to the groin and hamstring are generally acute injuries as well as severe blows to the upper thigh.

Hamstring Tear

There are three hamstring muscles, all three crossing the hip joint as well as the knee. Because they are biarticular (crossing two joints), and because they must coordinate knee and hip movements with the quadriceps during high-speed running, they are particularly susceptible to injury. Hamstring tears are serious, as running is seriously compromised and reinjury occurs frequently. New rehabilitation techniques developed by researchers at the University of Wisconsin utilized a program of progressive agility, trunk stability exercises, and icing to treat hamstring injuries, returning athletes to competition in 22 days, and there was no reinjury. Standard treatment involves static stretching, hamstring resistance exercises, and icing, typically returning athletes in 37 days, and has a poor record of reinjury. Extensive stretching of hamstring tears is not recommended. Question 41 presents weight training techniques to prevent hamstring tears.

Groin Muscle Tear

Due to the diagonal nature of hip movements in ice skating and soccer, adductor muscles (groin) in the thigh are susceptible to strain. Researchers at Lenox Hill Hospital in New York found that hockey players who had weak adductor (inside of thigh) relative to abductor (outside of thigh) muscles were 17 times more likely to sustain a groin strain. Strength and not flexibility were most related to injury. Research has shown that strengthening the groin muscles reduces the frequency of groin injury. Fatigue is also a factor, as ice hockey players suffer more groin injuries as the game progresses.

Thigh Contusion

A third acute injury to the hip area is a contusion to the upper thigh caused by a severe blow to the thigh, resulting in a hematoma. The reaction to such a blow is swift and should be treated immediately on the field with ice and rest but not elevation. Massage of the thigh exacerbates bleeding and should be avoided. One serious outcome of a severe contusion is acute compartment syndrome of the thigh. When pain and pressure continues following a contusion, and the athlete has trouble walking, prompt medical attention is in order. Even when treated properly on the field, the swelling can cause irreversible damage, renal failure, and possibly death. A second severe problem is the development of a calcium deposit in the muscle, sometimes resulting in myositis ossificans, a condition that might require surgery.

Hip Flexor Inflammation (Tear)

Hip inflammation and injury is a common overuse injury and involves the iliopsoas muscle, which consists of the psoas and the iliacus muscles. Flexion of the hip (raising the hip forward) is their main action, and it allows you to run forward and uphill. Hip inflammation is very common in cyclists and runners as well as those who do a lot of lunges, such as tennis and badminton players. Injury to these muscles is caused by overuse, but a direct blow can also injure as well. Early treatment is the answer to a quick recovery, and participants need to be aware of the symptoms including the following:

- Pain in front of the hip or groin
- Pain when going up stairs
- Pain when raising knee to chest
- A pulling sensation in upper thigh

Iliotibial Band Syndrome

Iliotibial band syndrome (ITBS) is another overuse injury originating in the thigh. The iliotibial (IT) band is a thick band of tissue on the outside of the leg that attaches to the top of the tibia (shin), providing stability to the knee and thigh. The tensor fasciae latae (TFL) muscle provides tension by attaching to the IT. When running (or walking), the end of the IT moves across the bony end (epicondyle) of the femur as the runner flexes and extends the knee. Occasionally, this back and forth movement causes friction and inflammation to the end of the IT, resulting in pain to the outside of the knee. The IT band is particularly active when standing on one leg, and since running has a period of one-legged support, running, especially long distance, is the principal cause of ITBS. Weak quadriceps, poor hamstring and TFL flexibility, and running behaviors such as running in only one direction around an oval or running on an uneven road but always on one side are problems. Stretching the TFL, ice, and rest are common short-term treatments to ITBS. Physical therapists may work on the biomechanics of running and footwear adaptations.

22. What are the most common injuries to the knee?

Stability of the knee is one of the most critical components of successful athletic performance. Most sports are played in a standing position, and excellent mobility is dependent on stable knees. But individuals who participate in supported sports, such as rowing and biking, and flex and extend their knees repeatedly also suffer knee injuries. Further, since knee injuries often have lifetime effects, quality of life can be compromised by knee injury in early life. The frequency of knee injuries can be reduced, and Question 47 provides specific information on how to improve stabilization and reduce injury.

The knee is the largest joint in the body, joining the large femur (thigh) bone with the two bones of the shin: the tibia on the inside and the fibula on the outside. Stabilizing the knee on each side are two ligaments: medial collateral ligament (MCL) on the inside that joins the femur to the tibia and the lateral collateral ligament on the outside that connects the femur to the fibula. The primary purpose of these two collateral ligaments is to provide stability from side to side. On the inside of the knee are two smaller ligaments, the cruciates. The anterior cruciate ligament (ACL) runs from the top of the tibia to the back of the femur, while the posterior cruciate ligament (PCL) runs from the top of the tibia to the front of the femur. The primary purpose of the cruciates is to provide stability forward and backward. On the inside of the knee joint are two articular discs (menisci). These cartilaginous discs aid in the absorption of force and provide stability of the femur on the tibia.

Very strong muscles support the knee in the front and back. In the front are the four quadricep (thigh) muscles that connect to the patella (knee-cap) to extend the knee. The patella then connects to the top and the front of the tibia via the patella tendon. Of the four quadricep muscles, only the rectus femoris (the kicker's muscle) is biarticular, affecting hip flexion as well as knee extension. In the back (posterior) are the three hamstring muscles. All of the hamstrings are biarticular, causing knee flexion and hip extension. The stability of the knee is dependent on the strength and coordination of the muscles as well as the strength of the ligaments. Of these structures, the tissues that are most vulnerable to injury are the MCL, ACL, menisci, patella and patella tendon, and the hamstrings. Unfortunately, many knee injuries involve injury to more than one structure such as tearing the MCL and the medial meniscus at the same time.

Medial Collateral Ligament Sprain

The MCL is frequently sprained, usually caused by a direct blow to the outside of the knee. Contact sports result in the most MCL injuries. The MCL can also be sprained by an uncontrolled landing such as coming down from a rebound in basketball. Fortunately, the MCL has excellent blood supply and normally responds well to nonsurgical treatment. Athletic trainers will often put a brace on the knee to reduce lateral movement during the early stages; rehabilitation starts early with the goal of restoring strength and flexibility, along with drills to improve mobility. Some MCL sprains come around in a week, but some require as long as eight weeks.

Meniscus Tear

Uncontrolled twisting of the knee, especially when the foot is planted and the body turns in the opposite direction, often results in a torn knee cartilage. A torn meniscus is usually treated with surgery (meniscectomy). Fortunately, with the advent of arthroscopic surgery, this surgery is not very invasive and recovery is relatively quick. Typical recovery is about four to six weeks, but there are reports of much shorter recovery periods. Unfortunately, since the surgery usually involves removing part of the torn cartilage, the knee loses some of its stability.

Anterior Cruciate Ligament Tear

A more serious knee injury is a rupture of the ACL. Even though the ACL is a fairly small ligament, its role in stability is crucial for high-functioning athletes. However, there are many instances when the ACL is torn and individuals go about their daily lives without compromise. One reason ACL tears are serious is that surgery is the normal treatment followed by a year of rigorous rehabilitation before returning to competition. Moreover, an initial ACL tear makes one more vulnerable to a second. Blocking and tackling in football is a common cause of ACL tears, but about 70 percent of ACL tears are noncontact injuries, happening during deceleration activities such as stopping, turning, and landing. Uncontrolled deceleration results in excess stress and subsequent tear of the ligament. Sports like soccer, basketball, and lacrosse that involve significant jumping and landing, often on one foot, are the primary problem sports. ACL ruptures often involve other tissues; the "terrible triad" is an injury to the ACL, MCL, and medial meniscus all at once. It is not unusual for an ACL tear to end one's competitive career.

Patella Injury

The patella, kneecap, suffers injury as well. The primary role of the patella is to improve the angle of insertion of the patella tendon. The patella has a V-shaped back that tracks up and down through a groove in the femur. An acute injury to the quadriceps may result in muscle weakness and displaced tracking, but individuals who have wider hips (usually females), flat feet, or knock-knees are at risk. Chondromalacia patella (or patella femoral syndrome) is the result of excess wear on the cartilage that covers the back of the patella. Chondromalacia is also called runner's knee and is one of the most frequent causes of knee pain.

The patella can also be fractured, primarily the result of landing directly on the unprotected kneecap. Direct contact can also cause dislocation of the patella, a condition in which the patella moves out of the joint (normally to the outside) and must be reduced. The knee tends to give way, and there is considerable pain; extending the knee is very limited. Patella dislocation can be treated surgically or in a more conservative nonsurgical protocol. Research is mixed on which is better, but most second dislocations are surgically treated. Unfortunately, about one-third do not regain their initial functionality. Treatment must involve high-quality rehabilitation with significant attention to strengthening the stabilizing muscles along with improved biomechanics while changing direction.

23. What are shin splints?

Shin splints has become a catchall phrase for pain in and around the inside of the tibia (shin). There are several sport-related problems that result in shin pain. The suggested label for the most common of these problems is medial tibial stress syndrome (MTSS). It is common in runners, and about 10–20 percent of runners will experience it in their career. Athletes in other sports, especially those in ballistic activities like football, soccer, basketball, and dance, are often susceptible. Other causes of shin pain are stress fractures and lower extremity compartment syndrome.

MTSS is an overuse injury. About 60 percent of all overuse injuries to the leg in runners are MTSS. Maladaptation is the basic cause. Bones and muscles normally remodel in a well-defined sequence, resulting in bones and muscles that are resistant to stress. Maladaptation occurs when the stress is either too great or when there is insufficient recovery. Maladaptation can affect the tibia when the bone becomes inflamed, causing periostitis, or muscles of the calf area can be strained resulting in pain to the inside of the tibia.

Training errors are the most common cause of MTSS, most commonly a sharp increase in intensity, especially in the early season of training when athletes are highly motivated to get in competitive condition. Running surface is another issue, when athletes may switch surfaces without a concomitant change in intensity. For example, switching from running on a track to running on grass will place stress on the lower leg that exceeds the familiar stress of the track. When switching surfaces, reducing volume and intensity should be considered. Athletes with inflexible or weak calf muscles as well as athletes who have weak trunk (core) muscles, resulting in excess pelvic girdle movement when running, are at greater risk of developing MTSS. Poor footwear can be another cause of MTSS.

Typically, athletes feel pain early in the run, which often diminishes during the run but returns upon cessation of training. If not treated, the condition worsens. Ice is a common therapy along with a modification in training. Reducing load by around 50 percent tends to help, along with cross training and pool running. Avoid hill running and changing surface during recovery. In some cases, orthotics are suggested but only prescribed by professional personnel. Typically, athletes should be able to return to full participation in four to six weeks.

Stress fractures are another product of maladaptation, and the tibia is frequently affected. The athlete feels burning and some discomfort along the shin. Running is painful, and as the condition worsens, walking is painful as well. Rest is the treatment for stress fractures, taking about six to eight weeks to recover.

Lower extremity compartment syndrome is occasionally confused with MTSS. The condition is more serious but less frequent. The muscles in the calf area are separated by fascia, forming four distinct compartments. If the muscles within a compartment tend to swell, the pressure increases, possibly leading to a dangerous condition, as blood supply can be impeded and nerve supply affected. This condition can be acute or chronic. A direct blow to the front of the shin injures those muscles in the anterior (front) compartment, causing swelling. One reason for shin pads is to resist anterior compartment syndrome. Compartment syndrome can occur in other areas, especially deep muscles in the back of the calf. Initial treatment is normally conservative involving icing and exercise reduction. However, severe compartment syndrome can involve surgery to release the tension (a fasciotomy). When the superficial compartments are affected, the recovery time is around 6 months, but deep compartments can take as long as 16 months to heal.

24. What are the most common injuries to the foot and ankle?

The foot is a marvel of complexity, the most human part of the anatomical structure. Not only does the foot account for about 25 percent of all the bones in the body, but the foot also has many ligaments, muscles, and tendons. Many of the muscles that move the foot and the toes are located in the calf, but some are intrinsic to the foot, allowing for infinite adjustments as we walk across uneven surfaces, run, jump, stop, and turn. Due to our upright stance, significant pressure is placed on the foot in almost all sports. There is no doubt that a healthy foot is an important key to athletic success. Unfortunately, injuries to the foot are fairly common and compromise athletic performance.

Ankle Sprain

Due to the nature of sports, it is no surprise that a sprained ankle is the most common injury in sports, accounting for approximately 17 percent of soccer injuries and 25 percent of basketball injuries. Ankle sprains often occur when landing from a jump, especially on one foot. About 80 percent of all ankle sprains are to the outside ligaments. Any ligament can be sprained. If the ligament more toward the front of the ankle is injured, the injury is not as serious as ligaments toward the bottom of the foot. Frequently mentioned by sport commentators is the high ankle sprain. This is actually a sprain above the ankle to the ligament that holds the bottom of the tibia and fibula together. This ligament takes longer to heal.

Question 48 discusses factors related to sprained ankles, including playing surface. Ice and a compression bandage are the typical treatments for a sprained ankle. Sometimes, the ankle is put into a cast or a splint for a brief period. Occasionally, an athlete will use one or two crutches in early stages, but treatment is encouraged soon after with functional rehabilitation. Typically, a Grade 1 (Question 9) injury takes one to two weeks to recover; Grade 2 takes about three weeks and Grade 3 up to eight weeks. Athletes are often taped or strapped while training and competing during the recovery phase.

Stress Fractures

Since stress fractures are the result of small forces being placed repeatedly over time, there is no surprise that the foot is susceptible. Athletes in running, basketball, volleyball, gymnastics, and cheerleading are especially vulnerable. Individuals who have weaker bones, especially women with irregular menses, are more vulnerable. Stress fractures often occur when there is an abrupt increase in training volume, leaving insufficient time for adaptation.

The metatarsals, the long bones that connect to the toes, frequently suffer stress fractures along with the calcaneus (heel). Pain is the specific symptom and is very specific to the injury site. Touching the specific area hurts. Walking or running increases the pain that eventually subsides upon stopping. A recent increase in activity along with specific pain is a symptom of stress fracture. Rest is the obvious treatment along with icing. Tylenol is the pain reliever of choice, as anti-inflammatory pain relievers like ibuprofen may increase the time for the bone to heal. It is important to place as little stress on bones of the foot during recovery, and some doctors will prescribe a walking splint. Most stress fractures of the foot and ankle will heal in four to six weeks. The fifth metatarsal, the bone on the outside of the foot, often takes longer to heal. During recovery, activities like swimming and cycling are recommended.

Plantar Fasciitis

Pain in the heel of the foot is normally caused by plantar fasciitis, inflammation of the fascia that runs from the inside of the heel over the bottom of the foot to the toes. This fascia is primarily responsible for the longitudinal (front to back) arch of the foot as well as for providing stabilization and shock absorption. Distance runners are particularly vulnerable, but anyone who spends considerable time on their feet can get plantar fasciitis. The exact cause of plantar fasciitis is unknown, but age and weight are factors. Individuals with flat feet are often more prone to getting plantar fasciitis. Some research suggests that plantar fasciitis is actually the cause of heel spurs.

One sign of plantar fasciitis is pain in the morning. People will often change the way they walk to relieve heel pain, often resulting in pain to other parts of the body like the knee or hip. The first step in treatment is to stop doing those things that cause pain. Ice and Tylenol will help along with wearing shoes that provide significant cushioning. Some individuals have success with night splints, a device that stretches out the calf muscles and Achilles tendon while sleeping. Improving the flexibility of the foot as well as massaging the bottom of the foot often helps. Orthotics prescribed by a foot specialist can take the stress off the plantar fascia. Most people will recover from plantar fasciitis after six months by providing their own conservative treatment at home. Ignoring the symptoms will result in a long period of problems.

Turf Toe

Turf toe is another cause of foot pain, an injury that has increased in frequency as a result of increased participation on synthetic surfaces with high friction. As a result, when athletes tend to stop quickly the shoe stops, but the foot inside the shoe tends to continue moving forward, rapidly extending the big toe. The rapid extension stretches the ligament under the toe, producing small tears. It's really a sprained big toe that can be very painful and debilitating. Like for most sprains, rest and ice are the treatment. A Grade 1 sprain may allow one to continue participating in a limited manner, but serious sprains often require weeks of recovery.

Achilles Tendon Injury

Problems occur in most sports involving running and jumping. This tendon is the strongest tendon in the body as it connects the two powerful calf muscles to the heel. Any landing from a jump will vigorously stretch the Achilles tendon. A subsequent contraction of the calf muscles places tension on the Achilles tendon. This rapid stretching and contracting places extensive stress on the tendon; little wonder that this tendon is injured and occasionally ruptured. The Achilles tendon can suffer acute tendonitis as well as long-term tendinosis. Acute tendonitis, often caused by an acute overload, is treated conservatively with a reduction in activity, icing, and a slow return to activity. A period of one to two weeks recovery is necessary, but return is usually successful. Long-term tendinosis is more problematic, requiring an immediate reduction in activity, especially uphill running and intense interval training. Eccentric muscle training (Question 41) has been successfully used to treat Achilles tendon problems.

A more serious injury to the Achilles tendon is a rupture. Achilles tendon ruptures are not uncommon in sports requiring intense jumping and landing. Intense pain, frequently accompanied by a snapping sound, and the inability to point one's toes are the immediate signs. Surgery is the recommendation, involving stitching the tendon back together, occasionally augmenting it with other tissues. A boot is normally worn for the first one to four weeks, dependent on the surgeon and the degree of injury. About four months of rehabilitation is suggested, during which time the range of motion, strength, and balance are restored. Specific training should continue as it takes at least a year for the tendon to return to normal.

Blisters

Blisters are not a serious foot injury, but they are painful and can ruin a long run or hiking trip. Athletic trainers report blisters as the most frequent problem treated in the training room during early seasons of practice. The best treatment for a blister is to not get one. A common problem is that athletes often get new shoes to start a new season, but shoes need to adapt. So bring along a second pair and switch when the first pair starts to present problems. Use this same technique with hiking boots before taking a multiday hiking trip.

25. What is a heat illness?

A heat injury or illness occurs due to the combination of exercise and heat. Heat illnesses can range from mild discomfort to death. Mild heat illnesses are very common, but about 600 deaths per year are related to heat. Significant changes in body temperature can result in illness or death. Hyperthermia (increased body temperature) is a significant problem for athletes since the body generates heat when exercising. The combination of the heat generated by exercise coupled with environmental heat stress overwhelms the body's ability to maintain normal temperature. This is particularly problematic during strenuous exercise as intense exercise produces even more heat.

Although football is the primary sport resulting in heat illness, exercise in any activity can cause heat problems. Two primary problems with football are that football practice normally starts in the heat of August and that the football uniform tends to prevent evaporation of sweat—one of the cooling mechanisms of the body. Compounding all of this is that for many years football coaches maintained the belief that fluid restriction was the best way to get their players in shape. There are numerous accounts of young athletes, particularly heavy ones, dying during football practice in the 1950s and 1960s.

Fortunately, research has shown the folly of this practice, and athletes are now allowed water during practice. Furthermore, various athletic federations have mandated an introductory training period, allowing athletes to acclimatize to exercising in the heat. During the training period, the athletes are often restricted from wearing the full football uniform. While these safe practices have reduced heat illnesses and death, some athletes still succumb to them. Question 49 describes how to reduce heat problems.

Besides temperature, humidity and radiation are problems as well. Not only do these environmental problems cause heat illness, but performance is also reduced. Blood normally returns quickly to the heart and lung, but when the body warms, blood tends to return to the heart through vessels close to the skin, thereby slowing blood flow return. Since the blood now takes longer to return to the heart, oxygen delivery to working muscles and brain is reduced.

Most texts describe four common heat illnesses from environmental stress and exercise.

Heat Exhaustion

Heat exhaustion is the most common heat illness, but it's a poorly defined syndrome. The typical symptoms are fatigue, weakness, dizziness, nausea, mild confusion, and muscle cramps. Heat exhaustion is primarily the result of excess fluid loss accompanied with the fatigue of exercise. Other than mild confusion, athletes do not suffer significant changes in mental status. Although heat exhaustion is not particularly serious, it indicates that the athlete does not have the ability to exercise vigorously in the heat.

Heat Syncope

Lightheadedness and occasional fainting are the symptoms of heat syncope, a fairly common heat illness. This condition is temporary and primarily the result of reduced blood flow to the brain. As mentioned, exercise in the heat results in reduced blood flow return to the heart and subsequently to the brain.

Exertional Heat Stroke

Exertional heat stroke (EHS) is serious. In the early twentieth century, only 20 percent of individuals with EHS survived. Now the survival rate is around 90 percent, but even this seems high. EHS is caused by a complete overload of the thermoregulatory system. Body temperature increases to around 104–105 °F. Excessive temperature leads to cardiac, liver, and kidney failure. Excess body temperature is a primary symptom, but mental confusion and disorientation are very common. Many times the athlete simply collapses. Athletes are often dry, but contrary to what many suggest, individuals with EHS often continue to sweat.

Muscle Cramps

Involuntary muscle spasms have long been associated with heat illness. Many texts list muscle cramps as a heat illness, suggesting that excess fluid and subsequent electrolyte loss leads to muscle cramps. However, studies have shown that individuals with muscle cramps often have the same electrolyte balance as individuals who do not cramp. The fact is that muscle cramps tend to be localized, affecting those muscles that have been fatigued. If muscle cramps were caused by electrolyte loss, one would expect that cramps would be more generalized. For example, individuals who have gone on a strenuous hike, especially one that is hilly, often get muscle cramps in their legs. Muscle cramps are probably due more to fatigue than dehydration. It just so happens that when a competitive season begins, athletes face heat illness and exhaustion at the same time.

Treating Sports Injuries

26. What is the typical therapy for different stages of healing for strains and sprains?

As discussed in Question 9, healing from sport injuries follows a defined sequence. Following recommended activities during each stage can reduce recovery time. In many instances, true healing will take longer than meeting the criteria to return to play (Question 35). Although the four stages of healing can be facilitated by therapy, the body will naturally follow the sequences of healing.

Bleeding

Bleeding is the first stage of healing. The acronym RICE is the common treatment to control bleeding: rest, ice, compression, and elevation. Of these, rest is probably the most important. In fact, rest is the most common form of treatment, as the body tends to heal itself as long as the stress is removed. Bleeding at the injury site causes swelling and pressure, often resulting in pain and reduced range of motion. During exercise, blood flow is enhanced as blood flow to muscles increases to deliver oxygen. Rest slows down blood flow. A common question is whether one can return to play after injury, especially a sport that is not overwhelming. The athlete is involved in the game, is motivated, and wishes to return. The athlete is also warm, and bleeding has not yet compromised movement. Although continued participation may not result in increased damage, the subsequent bleeding (and swelling) will be enhanced, resulting in more recovery time. Rest helps prevent excessive bleeding.

Reducing the temperature of the injured site slows blood flow. Icing is the common method of introducing coldness. Unfortunately, many do not have sufficient methods to cool the entire area. Many people do not have a good ice pack, or even ice. Frozen vegetables such as peas and corn work well. It's important to ice the entire site, so multiple packs should be used. To cool a torn hamstring, buy a bag of ice and put your leg on it. Icing for 24–48 hours is often recommended, using 15–20 minute sessions 3–4 times a day.

Compression also limits the flow of blood to a site. ACE bandages are the typical compression method, available at most pharmacies. These bandages come in different widths, so having more than one available is good. Simply wrap the bandage around the injured site, starting above the site and ending below it. Elevating the injured site slows blood flow, so keeping the injury site elevated is recommended throughout the day.

Inflammatory Phase

Inflammation happens very quickly following injury. This is the first stage of healing as injured tissue is removed from the injury site, allowing healing to begin. Acute inflammation ends in about seven days. During this time, there are a few practices the injured individual should do to promote healing and physicality.

- Control pain by taking Tylenol. Continue using ice to control pain. Avoid taking nonsteroid anti-inflammatory medications (NSAIDs) such as ibuprofen or aspirin.
- Begin restoring a range of motion by either active or passive exercises. Try to move the joints surrounding the injury without increasing the pain of the injury.
- In order to prevent atrophy, low-tension isometric (static) exercises can begin.
- Use novel exercises to maintain the fitness of other parts of the body.
- Maintain a high-quality diet.

Proliferative—Repair and Remodel

New materials such as collagen are beginning to repair the injury site. Exercise can begin with care, making sure not to reinjure. Pain-free strength training can begin, starting slowly and building. Use isotonic exercises (Question 41) involving fairly slow contractions and avoid ballistic activities like throwing and jumping. Engage the full range of motion and continue static stretching activities. Dependent on the extent of the injury, this period will last up to 21 days. During these last two stages, the use of heat prior to training is often helpful. Whirlpool baths and hot packs are typical methods; around 10–12 minutes is usually satisfactory. Icing after training is useful.

Maturation

The longest of the healing phases, maturation can take up to a year. Once the individual is comfortable with the ability to tolerate stress, progressive loading can begin. Slowly begin to increase the intensity and volume of activity. Continue to monitor the injury site, and if swelling or pain returns, slow down and allow some time for adaptation. Using heat during this training phase helps. Start performing ballistic activities like light throwing, kicking, and jumping. Warm up before all training, and remember that stretching activities, although recommended, are not a warm-up. Stretch at the end of the warm-up or following a training session. The goal of training in this stage is to replicate those activities one needs for successful participation in sport.

The following might be an example of a sequence one might use for a sprained ankle:

- Jogging in a straight line
- Doing toe raises on both feet
- Jogging faster
- Jogging and changing directions
- Doing toe raises on injured foot
- Balancing on one-dimensional balance board
- Hopping on both feet
- Running up a slight hill
- Running at a higher speed and changing directions
- Running and planting the injured foot and turning
- Hopping on injured foot
- Running with alternate hops on injured foot
- Sprinting at full speed
- Balancing on 360° disc
- Balancing on 360° disc on one foot

Functional rehabilitation is the key—training to perform all the activities one needs without pain. Care must be taken to move in a correct biomechanical manner without compromising other parts of the body. Rehabilitating in this manner reduces the incidence of reoccurrence.

27. What is the typical treatment for an overuse injury?

As discussed in Question 10, overuse injuries have increased significantly in all athletes including youth. Overuse injuries are not inflammatory problems—not acute injuries, but subtle. Typical symptoms of an overuse injury are as follows:

- Pain is gradual, often presented as an ache.
- Individual cannot remember when it started.
- Training and competition brings about stiffness.
- If continued, the ache and stiffness does not go away.
- Point tenderness develops.
- Swelling may occur.

Overuse injuries are degenerative changes, mostly to tendons. These injuries happen over time as a result of repetitive activities, usually activities that involve submaximal effort that can be repeated numerous times. Hitting a tennis ball over and over, cycling mile after mile, and overhand throwing are typical activities that result in overuse. The muscles repeatedly pull on the tendons; the tendons tend to degenerate, begin to ache, and get worse. Analgesics tend to lose their effectiveness.

Overuse injuries are the result of training errors, so it stands to reason that changing training is the first line of treatment. Question 39 provides suggestions on how to practice without overuse. Overuse injuries require a reduction in stress; rest is required. During the rest period, alternative training can be utilized, as it is unhealthy to stop exercise. Modifications can be made even in the same sport. Swimmers can swim different strokes, and baseball pitchers can play other positions. One key is to allow injured tissues to heal.

Normally, splints and casts are not recommended. Pain should diminish rather quickly, but there are no clear guidelines as to when one can resume training. Pain upon returning to activity is the best guideline to wait a bit longer. Once one can begin to resume their normal pattern of training, the recommendation is to start at about 50 percent of the preinjury workout and then build up at around 10 percent a week. Rushing beyond

10 percent a week will simply return one to the injury, requiring more rest and therapy. Keep in mind that tissues are being regenerated, and this takes time. When pain is encountered, decrease the workload and be patient.

Precede every exercise session by a gradual warm-up. This means performing related activities slowly, allowing the muscles and tendons time to increase internal temperature. Using warm hydrotherapy or hot packs tends to help, but these are not a substitute for the physical warm-up. Static and dynamic stretching should be used during each training session, but stretching is best done toward the end of a session. Icing can be used following activity. One therapy that has been utilized by some physicians is the injection of corticosteroids. There was a time when corticosteroid injection was routine, but this continues to be a debatable therapy. The effects are actually unknown, and some sources suggest that such treatments may actually be counterproductive.

A recent treatment that does seem very promising is the use of eccentric exercise (EE). As discussed in Question 11, eccentric contractions of muscles occur when the muscle is under tension but lengthening. Recently, studies have reported very good results for the use of EE to treat problems of the Achilles tendon, patellar tendon, and the lateral tendon of the elbow. The trick is to stress the injured muscle and tendon using eccentric training without excessive concentric training. For example, to primarily stress the quadriceps and the patella tendon, one can use a quad chair. Quad chairs are common to weight rooms where the participant sits and performs knee extensions. Lift the weight with both legs (concentric contraction of both legs) and then lower the weight with the injured leg (eccentric contraction). Raising the weight with both legs (concentric) will be relatively easy, but lowering the weight with only one leg should stress the eccentric aspect of contraction. Repeat about 10 times, rest, and then do two more sets of 10. If the activity is painful, reduce the weight, making sure the exercise is pain free. Slowly, increase the weight as strength increases. These EE exercises should be done on an alternate day basis. This kind of training can be utilized for many muscles and tendons such as the Achilles tendon, rotator cuff, and tendons of the elbow. For most individuals, professional help is recommended in order to perform these EE activities correctly.

28. What is the treatment for a concussion?

The first line of treatment for a concussion is to recognize that you have incurred one. A concussion occurs because of some form of blow. It is most often violent, but not always obvious. It could be a hit to the head in football, a fall, or going up for a header in soccer. Divers can get concussions when hitting the water. Qualified medical personnel diagnose concussions. Most concussions are temporary, especially if treated properly, but if one ignores the symptoms, they may continue to put themselves at significant risk. Although there is more publicity about the negative effect of concussions, study has shown that many are still not aware of the most common symptoms. Ignoring concussion symptoms makes a person particularly susceptible to future problems.

It is possible to receive a concussion and not know it. It is not unusual to see two individuals hit heads; one is left unconscious and the other seems OK. Why one person experiences a concussion and another person doesn't is unpredictable. Some signs and symptoms are subtle and take time to manifest. Some concussions cause unconsciousness, but most do not. Common symptoms include the following:

- Temporary loss of consciousness
- Headache—sometimes a feeling of pressure in the head
- Confusion or a foggy feeling
- Amnesia of the event
- Dizziness—may see stars
- Ringing in the ears
- Nausea and vomiting
- Slurred speech
- Slow response to questions
- Dazed

It is not necessary to have all of these symptoms to determine if you need a medical diagnosis. Further, other symptoms may be delayed, showing up days after the injury. These include the following:

- Fatigue
- Problems concentrating
- Irritability
- Problems sleeping
- Light and noise sensitivity
- Disorders of taste and smell
- Psychological problems such as depression

A concussion is an injury to the brain, and the primary treatment is to rest the brain. Exercising the brain during recovery is contraindicated; rest is the answer. This is often a problem for students and individuals involved in demanding jobs or work situations that are not flexible. People who have been concussed need to be given time to recover, and teachers and employers need to respect the time for recovery.

Until recently, it was suggested that people with concussions rest in a dark room with little stimuli. The problem with this treatment was that concussion symptoms actually increased. Removing outside stimuli left one focusing on their symptoms, actually increasing the awareness of symptoms. Mild stimuli actually allow one to attend to things other than symptoms. Activities during recovery should be mild; avoid complex problems, intense computer games, loud music, and bright light. Stay away from crowds. Eating well and taking naps are highly recommended.

Most concussion symptoms resolve within 7–10 days, but some take longer. During recovery, the following is recommended:

- Reduce screen time.
- Avoid bright lights and noise.
- Stay hydrated.
- Avoid sharp movements of the head and neck.
- Eat well.

One of the most important behaviors during concussion recovery is to avoid any additional injury. Activities like ice or roller skating and downhill skiing should be avoided. Mild swimming is OK, but do not dive in the pool. A problem for people living in northern climates is falling. Take extra care when going outside in winter. Wear some form of traction device under the bottom of shoes.

During recovery, it is important to seek medical help if there is a severe increase in symptoms, such as falling, unconsciousness, sudden intense headaches, or seizures. Following these guidelines usually allows one to fully recover and to return to play or their normal exercise program. Occasionally, some experience postconcussion syndrome resulting in long-term symptoms. Research has not identified why some get this.

With regard to return to plan (RTP) criteria, medical clearance should be obtained, and individuals should begin a gradual step-wise increase in activity once symptoms have resolved. Concussions often lead to an increased reaction time, putting one at additional risk. An individual should not return to play until they are fully functioning. If symptoms return, then additional recovery time is necessary, and activity should be stopped.

29. If you're injured while playing a school sport, how can an athletic trainer help with your injury? What about a strength and conditioning coach?

Almost all colleges and many high schools have certified athletic trainers who maintain athletic training rooms, attend practices and games, and care for the well-being of athletes. The National Athletic Trainers Association (NATA) began in 1950 and established the first certification program in 1986. The training and education of athletic trainers requires them to have a four-year undergraduate degree, specific courses in sports medicine, and an extensive amount of experience under the direction of certified athletic trainers. Athletic trainers generally coordinate the medical treatment of athletes, especially when it involves different individuals such as physicians, physical therapists, and strength and conditioning specialists.

More recently, many colleges now have strength and conditioning specialists. Some larger high schools have strength and conditioning trainers as well. The National Strength and Conditioning Association (NSCA) certify such individuals. The general certification is for a certified strength and conditioning specialist (CSCS), and recipients usually attach a CSCS label to their title. Individuals with a CSCS certification may work as personal trainers, but their certification is far more advanced than the certification necessary for personal trainers. CSCS individuals usually have a master's degree, and they would have satisfactorily passed a difficult exam and demonstrated their knowledge of training athletes.

Athletic trainers are the first line of evaluation and treatment for athletes. Unfortunately, many high schools do not have a full-time certified athletic trainer. Some have a part-time trainer who works at multiple schools, usually attending contests but with limited availability otherwise. Some schools simply rely on a coach or other personnel to assist with athletes who are injured. A uniform program of medical coverage does not exist.

Whether in high school or college, the athletic trainer generally operates out of a training room. Training rooms can range from a simple room with an exam table, an ice machine, and a treatment center for blisters and cuts to a sophisticated facility with x-ray, facilities for simple medical procedures, and numerous therapeutic modalities. During practices, athletic trainers are usually on call to respond to an injury on the field or in the gym. In sports where the injury rate is higher, athletic trainers can generally be found on the sideline during games, treating minor injuries such as cuts and abrasions, but primarily available for serious on-field injuries.

When an injury happens during a contest, the athletic trainer identifies the history of the injury, the seriousness of it, and whether the athlete can be moved. Thereafter, a return to play decision is made by the athletic trainer and possibly a physician who may be in attendance. Treatment is begun immediately. Thereafter, the athletic trainer plans therapeutic treatment. For serious injuries, athletic trainers normally arrange appointments to local physicians and are in contact with the physician. In addition, the athletic trainer usually confers regularly with the coaches to inform them of the athlete's status.

Once the athlete is capable of moving beyond the training room, they need to begin step-wise functional training. The goal is to return to the playing arena by regaining strength, movement, and proprioception, training the athlete to compete fully without additional risk of injury. The athletic trainer often organizes such training in conjunction with strength and conditioning specialists or coaches. Regardless of who is training the athlete, complete rehabilitation of the athlete must be conducted in the environment in which the athlete competes. If the athlete does not get out of the weight room to train, they are not ready to compete.

30. When should you see a physical therapist?

When a sport injury occurs, a program of rehabilitation helps one return to their preinjury condition. Mild sprains, strains, and bruises usually just require the immediate RICE procedure followed by a gradual return to activity. If one is careful to avoid reinjury, they can slowly return to full activity. In these situations, most do not seek outside help. But many injuries require more advanced rehabilitation, therapy, and modalities, most of which the public is unaware and is unavailable. Recovery from serious injury requires professional attention.

Individuals recovering from shoulder, knee, and elbow surgeries certainly require very specific therapy for recovery. Tendon surgeries often require long-term rehabilitation. Occasionally, individuals have lingering pain that does not abate. Therapy will often resolve the problem. As discussed in Question 27, many overuse injuries profit from eccentric exercises, but these exercises are difficult to employ, often requiring a therapist for design and assistance.

Individuals who play on organized school-sponsored teams will first encounter the certified athletic trainer hired by the organization. Some schools only have an athletic trainer who attends contests and is not available for longer-term care. Individuals who get hurt and are not affiliated with an institution are faced with finding their own support. Trying to design one's own therapy may compromise healing; professional help is required.

When injured, most people turn to their primary care physician. The physician will often send the patient to an orthopedic surgeon or to a physical therapist. Some states require that one should first get a prescription from their physician before seeing a physical therapist, but many states allow one to go directly to a physical therapist for diagnosis and treatment. Personal trainers are not an option, as they are not normally trained in rehabilitation.

Physical therapists are trained to diagnose injury and to restore physical function and mobility. They typically have a four-year degree followed by years of advanced training. They are licensed and can be found in a range of health-care settings. They take care of patients in all phases of healing, and patients can expect the following:

- Undergo a physical exam and evaluation to determine the extent of the injury.
- Receive a diagnosis, prognosis, and a plan of treatment.
- Receive treatment.
- Receive recommendations for at-home care.

Throughout this text, discussion has centered on the need to try conservative treatment of injury before undergoing surgery. Most sport injuries are treated conservatively and effectively. Physical therapy is conservative treatment, and most enjoy the following benefits:

- Avoiding surgery
- Achieving pain management with reduced need for opioids
- Having improved mobility and range of motion
- Regaining muscle strength
- Recovering proprioception and functionality

The cost of physical therapy varies with the area and the type of insurance one has. Typically, insurance companies allow a specific number of visits dependent on the injury. Frequently, one has to advocate for additional visits. The therapist is often involved in advocating for such visits. Following surgery, the surgeon can also advocate for adequate therapy.

Occasionally, the primary care physician will recommend that a patient see a physiatrist. Physiatrists are medical doctors who specialize in physical medicine and rehabilitation. Some specialize in sports medicine. Although most physiatrists do not perform therapy, unlike physical therapists they can prescribe medicine, imaging tests, and they can perform medical procedures. Physiatrists can diagnose sport injury and treatment and recommend therapists. Physiatrists often work closely with therapists to bring about coordinated care.

31. How do you select a physical therapist or a surgeon?

Choosing the right physical therapist or surgeon requires the patient to research, advocate, and decide what is best. Considering the fact that surgery and the recovery from surgery have lifelong effects, injured individuals need to make an informed decision on who operates on them and who helps them recover from injury. Occasionally, there are emergency situations when one needs immediate treatment in the emergency room, but most often the injured party has the opportunity to choose who treats them. When injured, take time, do the research, and choose the best person available for treatment.

Orthopedic surgeons are not all the same; they are not specifically trained in all surgeries. Although orthopedics is a medical specialty, the body is very complex, and one cannot expect surgeons to be skilled at operating on all joints or tissues. This is particularly true for hands and feet. Consider the fact that the foot contains 26 bones, 33 joints, and more than a hundred muscles, tendons, and ligaments. You do not want a surgeon who is an expert on knee replacement to operate on your foot. If you are having surgery on your rotator cuff, find a shoulder surgeon. Often, it may be more specific than just the joint. For example, there are knee surgeons who specialize in knee replacement. This surgeon may have a high rating but may not be the one to select for other knee surgeries, such as for an anterior cruciate ligament (ACL).

A frequent way to choose a surgeon is word of mouth. Find people who have had the same surgery. Ask specific questions: How successful was the surgery? Did the surgeon communicate well and follow up with the physical therapist? How difficult was it to contact the surgeon? Remember that you are not hiring a friend, but someone who will perform well, advocate for you, and follow up. Do not be afraid to get a second opinion. If you live in an area where there is a university, you may be able to locate surgeons who operate on the local athletes.

Rating systems exist on line for doctors. The "Directory of Resources" at the end of this book presents choices. Many people tend to lean more on how friendly the surgeon is. A friendly doctor is nice to have, but competency is more important. Hospitals are also rated, so take a look in the directory for hospital ratings. If a hospital has a low rating, infection may be an issue.

Complete recovery from an orthopedic surgery requires rehabilitation. Physical therapy is the main option, but physical therapists also specialize. Some are wonderful when dealing with back or neck injuries but less skilled when rehabilitating an ACL reconstruction. Several factors should be considered when finding a physical therapist.

Recommendations from physician are a good beginning. Keep in mind that when you are injured, you would want to return to preinjury condition. This means functional rehabilitation. Simply returning to pain-free range of motion is not enough. When going into a physical therapy facility, observe the demographics of the clientele. Is it mostly elderly individuals just trying to walk upright, or are there young people trying to get back to playing? What does the facility look like? If it is just a room of treatment tables, this is not the facility to train functional activities. Look for a facility that is more dynamic, that has people moving around on their feet. This is where therapists work, who will get you back to full activity. How does the physical therapist work with patients? Does the therapist do overlapping treatment, treat more than one patient at a time? Rehabilitation requires good form, and you need a therapist who is with you the entire time.

Rehabilitation takes time; it is not a rushed treatment. Time is needed for recovery, so be patient. But physical therapy should lead to positive results. Does the therapist appear frustrated that the treatment isn't working? If you are not getting better, it may be time to switch therapists. If you are doing everything you are supposed to do and not getting better, it may be time to change.

In general, the best predictors of successful recovery from an injury that requires surgery are the following:

- A surgeon who is specifically trained
- A surgeon who has performed that surgery many times
- A surgeon who wants to get you back to your preinjury state
- A physical therapy program that takes you from surgical recovery to functional rehabilitation
- A patient who is prepared to do the work necessary to recover

32. What are the most common surgeries to address sport injuries?

Surgery is not the first option for most sport injuries; conservative treatment is usually the first choice to return individuals to their previous level of activity. But some sport injuries will not heal without surgery. Tissues such as the anterior cruciate ligament (ACL) and severely torn tendons require surgery. New surgery techniques, pain management procedures, and expert rehabilitation now make surgery a less painful and easier option. Most surgeries are now performed arthroscopically, providing a minimally invasive approach to repair damaged areas.

Meniscectomy or Meniscus Repair

A meniscectomy is a removal of all or part of the meniscus in the knee. When the meniscus is torn, turning and lateral movements are painful. Occasionally, a piece of the meniscus floats around within the knee and dislodges the knee, making it seem as if the knee joint is out of place. This is very uncomfortable but usually resolves. When the meniscus is removed, the pain of twisting and turning movements is removed. On the negative side, the removal of all or part of the meniscus reduces cushioning and stability. Almost all meniscectomies are outpatient procedures. The patient is anesthetized with either a general or a local anesthetic. The leg will be bandaged, and patients are encouraged to ice and elevate for the first two days. Crutches are normally provided but are only necessary for a short time. Recovery can be as little as three weeks and up to six months dependent on the degree of tear.

Anterior Cruciate Ligament Repair

ACL repair is more difficult with a longer recovery. In most cases, ACL surgery does not happen immediately after injury but after a period of physical therapy to improve mobility and strength. The surgery is a replacement of the ACL with other tissues of one's own body. The typical reconstruction is to replace with a section of the patella tendon. Occasionally, if the individual already has patella tendon problems, pieces of the hamstring tendon are used. The decision of which tissue to use is normally made by the orthopedic surgeon. Like the recovery for meniscectomy, using ice and elevation is very important. Walking on crutches is normally required for a week or two, but rehabilitation will start immediately after surgery. Full recovery usually requires about a year.

Rotator Cuff Surgery

Rotator cuff surgery is normally conducted only after extensive physical therapy. Surgery to the rotator cuff is not the first choice, as there is the risk of considerable damage to the overlying muscles and intensive scarring. Rotator cuff surgery is either arthroscopic or through traditional open repair. The arthroscopic method is less invasive and results in less damage.

Rotator cuff surgery may involve one or all three of the following:

• Debridement—removal of loose fragments within which the rotator cuff muscles move
• Smoothing—making room so rotator cuff tendons and muscles can function without being pinched (impingement)
• Stitching—torn tendons are stitched back together and to the humerus

Most patients stay one night in the hospital. Usually, the injured arm is placed in a sling that holds the arm in a flexed position. The sling is often worn for around five weeks, but rehabilitation begins soon after surgery to regain motion. Early rehabilitation is rather mild, giving time for tissues to heal. Complete recovery from this surgery takes months, and the shoulder will probably not return to preinjury status.

Separated Shoulder Surgery

The end of the collarbone (clavicle) attaches to the acromion process of the shoulder blade (clavicle) by the acromioclavicular ligament (AC ligament). When this ligament is completely torn, surgery is the choice. Several surgical techniques are used to reconstruct the AC ligament. Following surgery, a sling is normally worn for about four weeks. After the first week or two, some mild exercises can begin, and full range of motion usually takes six to eight weeks. An extensive rehabilitation period will then follow, but it will take about eight months to recover from this surgery.

Tommy John Surgery

When the UCL (the ligament on the inside of the elbow) is torn or deteriorated, the ability to throw or hit overhand is seriously compromised. It is called Tommy John surgery because the first successful reconstruction of this ligament was done on the baseball pitcher Tommy John. Tommy John surgery is quite common with a success rate from 85 to 92 percent. This surgery is generally an outpatient surgery lasting 60–90 minutes. A tendon from another part of the body such as the palmaris longus tendon (a forearm muscle) is used to replace the torn ligament. Usually, a 3–4 inch incision is made to clean out the joint and remove damaged tissues. Holes are drilled in the two bones the original ligament is attached to, and the graft tendon is threaded through these holes and secured by sutures, buttons, or screws.

Rehabilitation normally follows three phases, each varying in time dependent on how fast tissues heal.

- Immediately after surgery, the elbow is secured in a brace at a fixed angle. The main goal during this time is to protect the joint. Physical therapy involves using one's wrist and fingers and some shoulder and biceps work.
- The second phase starts in one or two weeks, when one can start moving their elbow to restore range of motion.
- The third phase starts about a month after surgery. The patient will stop wearing a brace, regain complete range of motion, and start strengthening. Complete recovery takes about a year.

Patella or Achilles Tendon Repair

Both the patella and Achilles tendons are susceptible to rupturing. Surgery is typically outpatient, during which time the surgeon stitches the tendons back together. In some instances, tendons are taken from other parts of the body to supplement the original tissue. Occasionally, bone may be pulled away, which needs reattachment. Although the tissues will always be somewhat compromised, surgery is generally successful.

33. What if I continue to injure myself and need more surgeries?

In Michael Sokolove's book *Warrior Girls*, he tells the story of Amy Steadman. *Parade* magazine called her "the best of the best," as she left high school and headed off to play soccer at the University of North Carolina. Amy's dreams of a soccer career were never realized. By age 20, she had undergone five knee surgeries. She had to give up the sport; she walked with an inflexible gait, somewhat like an older woman. Amy was a warrior, willingly going through surgeries and relentless in her rehabilitation, but regardless of her tenacity, she will have to contend with a serious knee problem the rest of her life.

The question one needs to ask is not whether to get surgery but whether to continue to play after surgery. Surgery reduces pain, often allowing one to continue sport. There is little doubt that the original injury and surgery increases risk. For example, one study found that one is six times more likely to tear their ACL after surgery. One might ask if it was worth it. The answer is unknown, but young people who suffer such injuries need to understand that they are putting themselves at great risk when they return to play. So many youth work hard during their early days to make the team; quitting seems wrong. Teammates want you to return; many parents and coaches support a return to competition. Returning is admirable, heroic. But what if you return to competition and the same injury occurs? You may be left with a knee or shoulder that never works right again. Your heroism is forgotten as you look ahead to 50 or 60 years of a compromised joint.

Sportscasters frequently point out football and basketball players who have suffered ACL reconstruction. Tear your ACL; get it fixed and return to competition. But the players on television are a very small minority. While they are playing at risk, they are also making a lot of money. For them, it may be worth it. But the vast majority of ACL reconstructions are done on athletes with no athletic future. No monetary awards exist.

Obviously, the knee is not the only joint that may receive repeated injuries. Rotator cuff surgeries are another problem. This is a complicated surgery that is not always successful. In fact, rotator cuff surgery will not return the shoulder to 100 percent function. Studies show that the odds of success are about 95 percent when the torn tendon(s) are small, but retear rates for large tears are about 20 percent. The probability of a retear is high; it seems wise not to attempt to return to the situation that caused the original injury.

Tommy John surgery has become much more frequent, especially among teenagers. The success rate of Tommy John surgery is fairly good, ranging from 80 to 85 percent, but this also means that 15–20 percent are not successful. Success is determined by whether the individual returns to compete, not whether the pain of a torn ligament is removed. There is simply not enough data on this surgery to determine a reinjury rate. Regardless, repeating this surgery is unusual, and the success rate is probably lower.

There is little question that if you tear your Achilles tendon or your patella tendon, you have to have it fixed. These injuries, if not repaired, lead to serious ambulatory problems. You cannot walk normally, and running is impossible. The rate of re-rupture on the Achilles tendon is about 1.7–5.6 percent. Tearing either of these tendons a second time will result in a compromised future.

People who tend to have had repeated sport injuries can enjoy a lifestyle of physical activity. Injury should not result in one giving up sport or exercise; there are alternatives. Finding new activities is a challenge, but one that can be enjoyable. If you've had a serious injury, find an activity that does not stress the original injury. Learn something new; regardless of your injury, you can find a suitable alternative exercise.

Suffering a serious injury and surgery, especially at a young age, is tough. No one wants to give up his or her sport, but going through a long life with a painful and compromised body is tougher. The decision is not an easy one, and it is a decision that must be taken seriously. Use resources you trust to make the right decision. A lifetime of exercise and sport adds greatly to one's quality of life. The joy of participation can always be there, but the more we hurt ourselves, the harder it gets.

34. Why is rehabilitation so important?

When a person gets injured, the primary goal is to recover from that injury, to return to the playing field or gym. Treatment is the first step, but treatment is only the beginning of recovery; without the next step, rehabilitation, the injured person will return to activity with reduced function and an increased tendency toward reinjury. Often overlooked, rehabilitation is the process to recover full function, the transition from injury to the resumption of performance. Rehabilitation requires adherence, diligence, and a positive attitude toward recovery; rehabilitation can be quite tough, lasting from a few weeks to a year. Rehabilitation should have two purposes: regain preinjury level of physicality and prevent future injuries.

Rest is the first stage of treatment, but rest also means inactivity, a condition that results in muscle atrophy, the reduction in muscle mass. Studies have shown that atrophy starts soon after immobility. Extreme examples of rest are when a limb is placed in a cast or sling to reduce motion. Anyone who has been in a cast for an extended period can attest to the extreme state of muscle atrophy that occurs. Removing the cast reveals a limb that is severely wasted, a limb that is stiff and significantly smaller than the uninjured limb.

Atrophy is only part of the problem as disuse results in a stiffer limb and a muscle system that is unused to working. Rest compromises the range of motion of joints. Inactivity also affects muscular control. Rehabilitation requires not only a rebuilding of muscle mass but also a return to the neurological control one enjoyed prior to injury.

Rehabilitation should involve activities that restore strength, flexibility, and endurance of muscle and connective tissue, but it should also include activities designed to restore the neurological control of movement to regain the synchrony of muscle contraction and relaxation that is necessary for powerful and efficient movement. Depending on the injury, as well as the activities in which one engages, the exact steps to recovery will vary. Each sport or activity has its unique requirements, and rehabilitation must address this uniqueness.

Resistance training is critical in rehabilitation and normally begins with low-intensity training. The purpose of this training is to regain strength as well as endurance of the muscle. Resistance training also begins the adaptation of tendons and ligaments, to restore balance and flexibility. During the early training, it is recommended that one uses unilateral (one limb at a time) activities. Monitoring is very important, making sure the tissues are not overstressed. Soreness and discomfort should be expected, but pain is the manifestation of a problem.

Resistance training also has a neurological effect since one is learning how to recruit muscles to overcome resistance. To enhance neurological training, resistance training should become more complicated, moving toward more bilateral exercises and exercises that require more balance. Free weights (as discussed in Question 41) require more balance and coordination. Injury usually results in some deconditioning of the whole body, so rehabilitation should involve all of the body. In particular, muscles of the trunk, the core, require training. Virtually all movements of the body require forces transmitted through the core. Rehabilitation is whole body training.

In addition to resistance exercises, one needs to engage in various exercises and drills that require balance, coordination, and agility. Drills should progress from slow to fast, eventually resulting in high-speed activities replicating impending participation. Since systematic and regular training is necessary for adaptation, adherence to a rehabilitation schedule is a key to success.

Finally, some individuals may need psychological support. Depression is not uncommon. When an injury occurs, there is usually immediate support; people are empathetic, but rehabilitation is often a lonely activity.

Further, fear of subsequent injury and fear of the future are frequent hurdles. Fear brings about inhibition, a state that compromises movement.

Question 35 discusses return to play criteria, but returning to play is dependent on a planned, fairly conservative sequence of progressively intense activities designed to replicate all of those activities one might encounter upon returning to full participation. During rehabilitation, minor setbacks are common, but they should not be considered failure. The body will heal.

35. When can I return to participation?

When to return to play often determines the success of the rehabilitation program. An early return places the athlete at additional risk, a risk greater than for the non-injured athlete. Since reinjury results in increased recovery duration, a conservative approach is best. The athlete must be ready to play at a speed that equals the preinjury level. In general, you should be able to answer several questions positively.

Am I Pain Free When I Make the Movements Necessary to Play?

Athletes certainly know when something hurts, so if the injury still hurts, then rehabilitation is not complete. But athletes must test themselves under playing conditions. This doesn't mean that one must play a full game or match but that they have participated at a fairly high level. If one does this while participating fully and are pain free, then they can answer this question positively.

Am I as Strong and Powerful as I Was when I Started?

Strength, power, and muscle endurance can all be measured. Athletes who play on organized teams often undergo performance tests prior to the start of a season. Strength and power is not that difficult to measure. However, strength and power during performance are less easy to measure, so it is necessary to determine this during play. No test really emulates what is required during competition. One recommendation is to measure the injured limb against the healthy limb. Both limbs should be equal. Can you hop across the floor on the injured leg as easily and well as the healthy leg? Is your injured shoulder equal to the healthy one? If the answer to these questions is not positive, you are not ready to return to full-speed activity.

Do I Have the Same Endurance while Playing as
I Did before Injury?

Endurance while playing can only be measured while performing one's sport or activity. When returning to play, most athletes do not have the endurance to play an entire contest. A good way to control this is to reduce the duration of activity. This means playing fewer tennis games, only playing half of a basketball game, or gradually increasing the duration as fitness returns. Once fatigue starts, it is time to take a break. Fatigue causes injury.

Has My Speed and Agility Returned to Preinjury Status?

Many athletic coaches and strength and conditioning coaches test their athletes using agility and speed tests. Repeating these tests post-injury helps to provide good return to play criteria. However, athletic competition is so complex that no test really emulates all of the movements encountered in a sport. For example, your knee may feel fine during sprinting or lifting weights, but the turning and surprised movements required to play squash or badminton can only be tested on the squash or badminton court.

For most athletes, intuition must not be overlooked. Athletes know their bodies; they know how sport feels and how their bodies react to the stress of performance. Athletes need to trust their intuition, to answer the question "Am I ready?" Athletes know when they are ready and must trust themselves before relying on the opinion of others.

Am I Confident That I Can Perform?

Athletes who have been on the sideline for a while often have mixed feelings about returning. Athletes often report concern that they are not going to be able to perform at their preinjury level. Returning to sport slowly will help with confidence. Athletes should not return to activity and expect to repeat exactly what they did prior to injury. One important aspect is that the athlete should have autonomy regarding when to return. This means that the athlete is the eventual person to make the decision, not the athletic trainer or coach. By returning slowly and following one's own intuition, the athlete will regain confidence, reduce fear of failing, and make a recovery.

Rehabilitation should not end once an athlete has returned to play. This is especially true for muscle strains as studies have shown that while an athlete might have regained their functional ability, the muscle fibers have not returned to their preinjury condition. Finally, there are times when the athlete should not return. The long-term risk may simply be too great. There is no perfect answer for this situation, but athletes need to understand the risk of future participation. This is very difficult for individuals who have a strong identification as an athlete, for an athlete who has spent years working hard to succeed. Therapy is often recommended and helpful.

Preventing Sport Injuries

36. Can sport injuries be prevented?

Millions of high school and college athletes play sports almost daily. Millions more exercise and play sports for fitness and recreation. Although the benefits of regular exercise are unequivocal, participation in sport can result in injury, an injury that might have lifelong effects, pain, and considerable expense. Injury is a common reason that people may stop their exercise program. In competitive athletics, injury can affect the success of the athlete and the team and end careers. Fortunately, proper training and behavior can significantly reduce the incidence of injury. Questions 43–48 cover specific training methods to reduce injuries to select parts of the body.

One key to reducing sport injuries is to understand how they occur in the first place. If one knows how injuries tend to occur, the etiology of the injury, they can then utilize specific training activities to address the problem. Indeed, activities designed to reduce injury are often exercises that also improve performance. High-performing athletes all utilize injury prevention activities in their training. Such activities are not a waste of time but a key to success.

For example, in Question 47 research is presented discussing how most injuries to the ACL are not the result of direct contact, but occur during deceleration activities. When athletes stop, turn, or land in an uncontrolled fashion, considerable stress is placed on the ACL. Athletes can be

Table 4 Modifiable Variables in Injury Prevention

Warm-up
Protective equipment
Conditioning
Technique
Overuse
Fatigue
Nutrition
Excess pressure to win
Muscle strength imbalance
Playing surface
Playing opponent
Illegal play

trained to stop, turn, and land in a more stable way, therefore reducing the incidence of ACL injuries.

In the sports medicine literature, a common discussion is about a list of variables related to injury. Many variables are present but out of the control of the participant. Table 4 lists those variables over which the participant has some control.

Warm-Up

Studies on the efficacy of warming up have been around since 1945, when Swedish researchers discovered that when muscle temperature increases, the ability to perform fast activities improves. Warm-up improves performance since the physiological effect of warm-up allows muscle to contract and relax faster, reduces stiffness, and improves blood flow to muscle. Warm-up also allows one to psychologically prepare. Research has shown that second-half injuries in football can be significantly reduced with only a three-minute warm-up following half-time.

A related warm-up is best, a warm-up that replicates what the demands of participation will be, starting slowly and increasing the warm-up activity. Occasionally, an athlete cannot perform a related warm-up, so a more general warm-up period should be conducted, consisting of calisthenic and other activities to warm the body. Some athletes insist on static stretching prior to competition. Although the efficacy of static stretching prior to performance is still debated, athletes need to know that static stretching does not warm muscles and should be conducted along with true warming activities.

Protective Equipment

The athletic associations that supervise sport normally mandate the type of protective equipment required for participation in organized athletic competition. The National Collegiate Athletic Association (NCAA) in college competition and high school sport federations govern sport and determine the protective equipment. Two problems exist within these programs: protective equipment should be worn in practice as well as games, and all players should have the same protective equipment. Second team players should not receive inferior or hand-me-down equipment.

In the recreational world, the primary protective piece of equipment is the helmet. Individuals participating in bicycling, downhill skiing, whitewater boating and rafting, and rock climbing need to wear a helmet, a helmet that is designed for the sport in which they participate. In other words, do not use a rock climbing helmet for cycling.

Conditioning

It is somewhat of a paradox that one way to prevent injury is conditioning (training), yet a common reason for injury is training error. Conditioning prepares an individual for competition, and an undertrained athlete is clearly susceptible to injury. Conditioning promotes fitness and health, yet too much training results in overuse injuries, overtraining syndrome, and burnout. In top-level competition, a fine line separates an athlete from being overtrained to peaking for top performance.

A common problem in training is whether one is specifically trained. Let's say that you are a regular jogger, a successful jogger, easily running 15 miles a week. When jogging, you run about 7 mph. Now your neighbor convinces you to join in the weekend touch football game. You go out for a pass, catch it, and start sprinting toward the goal line. You're now running 17 mph; you're not prepared for intense running. Snap goes your hamstring. You may be in great shape, but you are not prepared to play touch football.

Overuse

Throughout this text, numerous injuries have been identified as overuse injuries. A belief that "more is better" is one problem. Question 39 discusses how to improve performance while reducing the frequency of overuse injuries.

Fatigue

Athletes frequently experience transient fatigue, the fatigue brought about from extensive repetitions without rest. Athletes can also experience cumulative fatigue, the fatigue resulting from extensive training, poor sleep, and inadequate nutrition. As discussed in Question 41, the integrity of joints is highly related to muscle strength and coordination. As individuals repeatedly perform the same task, muscles tire and are not capable of maintaining their normal support. Also, coordination is reduced with fatigue, making individual joints more vulnerable. Athletes need to be in top shape to perform and to practice without the excessive fatigue that makes an athlete more injury prone.

Excess Pressure to Win

Athletes who develop a "win at all cost" mentality place themselves at greater risk of injury. Playing with an injury or while sick places an athlete in jeopardy. Athletes might attempt a stunt such as in gymnastics, cheerleading, or skiing for which they are not prepared. Many times, the excess pressure to win comes from external sources like coaches or parents. Certainly, athletes enter a competition with the desire to win, to do their best, but all athletes will lose at some point. Regardless of the level of competition, athletes need to take care of themselves, to take a position that they are not going to put themselves at risk.

Muscle Imbalance

Imagine playing a sport from an early age during which you only turn your body in one direction. This is true of golfers and often for rowers. Individuals in such sports need to participate in training activities designed to develop the entire body. Question 41 discusses how to do strength training to develop symmetry.

Playing Surface

In 1965, the first indoor dome stadium, the Astrodome, was opened in Houston, Texas. The original version of Astroturf was fairly hard and had greater friction than grass. Athletes complained that hitting the ground hurt more. Since then, competing companies have developed many versions of artificial surface. The result is a surface that more resembles, but is not equal to, grass. Artificial surfaces still have some of the original problems, but there is also the benefit of uniformity. In addition, since artificial surfaces can be plowed, athletes in northern climates can train during the winter, possibly making them more conditioned for competition.

Grass is a great playing surface, but without excellent maintenance, uneven spots develop. Research in Australia showed that when soccer fields are watered regularly throughout the season, injury is reduced. Footwear should match the playing surface. Does the athlete have the right shoes for the surface?

Playing Opponent

There is no question that athletes should be competing against athletes of their own ability and size. One of the worst practices in college football, and some high schools, is that good teams composed of bigger and faster athletes schedule inferior teams at the beginning of the season. The better teams gain experience, but the inferior teams place their athletes at increased risk as they are faced with opponents who are decidedly larger and faster.

Unequal opponents are not that unusual in youth sports. Some youth teams are poorly supported while others have better equipment, trained coaches, and more athletes. Many youth sport organizations develop rules to reduce substantial differences. Such a practice should be developed across the board in youth sport.

Illegal Play

Many of the rules in sport are written to protect athletes from injury. Late or out-of-bound hits in football are illegal, yet they still happen. Various blocks in football are illegal, and rules are written to protect basketball players while jumping. Due to the excessive and serious injuries to football quarterbacks, recent rules have been written to provide additional protection. Certainly, many injuries related to illegal play are simply accidental, part of the excitement of the game, but some athletes do not play fair and cause serious injury. Everyone involved in sport should work tirelessly to enforce legal play.

Interestingly, the recent interest in the long-term effects of head injuries has finally gotten the attention of football officials. Using one's head and helmet as a weapon is now illegal. It has taken years to recognize the imprudence of using the head and helmet as a weapon. Although it is well known that illegal play can cause injury, it is imperative that all levels of sports—players, coaches, officials, and administration—work to insist on illegal play.

Since sport injuries can be so devastating, individuals involved in sport at all levels should be aware of how to reduce the incidence of injury. The incidence of sport injuries can be reduced, but it must be part of all sport programs. Taking time to utilize injury reducing strategies is not wasted time.

37. How do I start a fitness program without hurting myself?

A major goal should be to develop a fitness routine that you can do all the time. It is far easier to stay in shape than to get in shape. Maintaining fitness is one key to avoiding injury since your body has already adapted to exercise. This doesn't mean you have to be in tip-top shape all the time; just don't let yourself become completely sedentary.

Starting a fitness program is one of the best things you can do for your health. Regular physical activity results in a host of well-researched benefits. Other than the usual health improvements, such as improved cardiovascular health, people who are more fit can experience an enhanced quality of life. Being fit allows you to participate in more activities without excessive fatigue. Activities become enjoyable rather than exhaustive, allowing you to participate without a loss of vitality. But a sport injury can rob you of vigor, reversing gains you have made and requiring you to start over again. You should adopt a fitness plan that works, is doable, and doesn't hurt you.

What does it mean to train? How does the body change? You adapt. Exercise presents stress to the body, a stressor that when systematically applied results in adaptation. Furthermore, adaptation is specific to the stress being applied. For example, if you perform a low-intensity but long exercise activity you gain endurance. Your heart and lungs improve in function, blood flow increases, and endurance increases. If you perform a high-intensity but brief activity such as lifting a heavy weight, you get stronger. The nervous system learns to exert more force and muscle fibers get stronger. Adaptation is specific to the stress.

"One size fits all" doesn't work in fitness. One person's activity is often unsuitable for another. Only you know how an exercise feels; let your own intuition judge how difficult an exercise is. Attempting to model someone on television who appears to exercise for a living is a mistake. Find your own rhythm; listen to yourself.

How should exercise feel? Many exercise trainers suggest taking heart rate, and many companies make money by selling watches or heart rate monitors. If you're the kind of person who likes to quantify their exercise program, go ahead, but it is a lot easier to simply tune in to your symptoms. What is your perceived exertion? What is your body telling you?

Exercise should feel "somewhat hard." What should "somewhat hard" feel like? You should feel some exertion; breathing should be noticeable, but you should not be gasping for air. You should be able to talk but probably not for long interrupted periods. You should not be able to sing. You should feel some strain, but you should also feel good, enjoying the physical aspect of your being. Listening to your body is a skill you can develop, an easy way to gauge intensity, a safe way to exercise without hurting yourself.

Getting Started

Don't make it complicated. There's so much written about getting fit that you're not sure what to do. Almost anything you do will work; just make sure you don't do so much you get hurt. You are just beginning, so you want to start cautiously and progress slowly. If you already have an injury or a medical condition, consult your physician or physical therapist for advice. Initial exercise is going to result in some soreness, but make sure you know the difference between soreness and the pain of injury. Soreness is more generalized while the pain of an injury is more localized, a more stabbing pain. You can ignore soreness but not the pain of injury. When this occurs, try to determine the cause and choose another activity; repeating the activity that caused the initial pain will just make it worse.

Should You Get a Personal Trainer? Join a Gym? Take a Class?

Personal trainers are often a good choice to get you going, especially if you are a true novice. But be careful if the trainer does not seem to tune in to you. Many trainers are quite fit and do not really understand how an exercise novice feels. But you need to learn to exercise on your own, without oversight. Joining a gym provides the variety that most need. A gym membership is also a commitment, a decision to get started, a motivator. Classes can be fun, but make sure you take one appropriate to your fitness. Stay away from the "boot camp" approach.

What about Web-Based Exercises?

There are a lot of advertisements for indoor cycling training. These always show superbly fit individuals working very hard. Is this the best exercise for you? At some point, this may work for you, but you need to know if you even like indoor cycling. There are some very strenuous workouts you can find on the Internet, but the big problem is that these programs are not tailored for you. Trying to imitate some super-fit person on your computer screen will probably be too stressful.

What Is the Best Aerobic Exercise?

The best exercise is probably the one you will do and enjoy. All aerobic activities have their inherent strength and weakness. Many people love jogging, but jogging is not a very good activity for people who are overweight or have knee or foot problems. People who are challenged with body weight will find supported activities like biking, swimming, or rowing less stressful. Walking is a great activity for almost everyone; all you need is a good pair of supportive footwear. Try walking in different environments and not always on paved surfaces. Walking across a field or on a trail provides a change in scenery and also improves stability. Each step on a trail requires you to stabilize your foot and body.

It is not necessary to limit yourself to only one activity. Mixing it up is OK, but you still need enough specific stress to adapt. Doing a different activity each day of the week is not a good idea. Try to have fun. An exercise partner of similar fitness is a great idea. If you can find someone, make it a priority.

What Should an Exercise Session Include?

Let's say you joined a gym and want to do a workout. One plan is to break up your workout into sections.

- Aerobic section: Most gyms have multiple aerobic stations. Walking or running on a treadmill, exercising on an elliptical, or cycling are easy and good choices. You probably don't need a warm-up for these activities.
- Anaerobic section: This section is a period of calisthenic and strength exercises. Alternate between pushing and pulling exercises to develop symmetry.
- Cool down: Since you should already be fairly warm from the previous activities, now is a good time to do some flexibility exercises.

The Non-gym Approach

You don't need a gym to work out. In fact, many people create their own personal exercise program with excellent results and never set foot in a gym. Who needs a gym to take a walk or a hike? Take a bike ride—no gym required. Need to do some stretching? Lie down on your living room rug. Buy a foam mat. Strength training? Expensive chrome resistance machines not required. You can use your own body weight to apply resistance. Buy a few dumbbells and kettle balls. These are a lot cheaper than a gym membership. Play tennis, squash, or racquetball. Walk and play golf—18 holes is around 6 miles of walking.

How Much Exercise Is Enough?

A common recommendation is to perform moderate exercise for about 30 minutes a day, five days a week. This amounts to 150 minutes a week. This is a fairly easy goal, but one that requires some planning. Fortunately, research has shown that you can break up the 30 minutes into smaller units. If you are truly a novice at fitness, anything you do will help. In addition to a moderate exercise, some strength exercises should be planned at least twice a week.

The 10 Percent Rule

As you get fitter, you are going to want to increase your volume. "Fitness begets fitness," as one trainer said. Herein is one of the problems that might result in injury. One way is to use the 10 percent rule; increase no more than 10 percent a week. So if you're jogging a mile a day, just go up to 1.1 miles. Your body will adapt to this new mileage, and the increased strain will not overload your ability to adapt.

Fitness Is Not a Job

One key to a successful fitness program is to build it into your normal day. Try to make fitness a typical part of your day, just like eating or bathing. There may be days when you don't feel like exercising. You may be tired or stressed from work, and you just need to rest. Here's when you need to listen to yourself. A fitness program should not rule one's life. It is not a job; it's just one of the good things to add to your life. Avoid exercise obsession. A moderate fitness program that you find enjoyable is the key. Stay fit all year and avoid injury. Get yourself in shape and stay there; be satisfied.

A major goal should be to develop a fitness routine that you can do all the time. It takes a bit more effort in the beginning, but it is far easier to stay in shape than to get in shape. Also, maintaining fitness is one key to avoiding injury since your body has already adapted to exercise. Getting in and out of shape throughout the year is a recipe for problems. This doesn't mean you have to be in tip-top shape all the time; just don't let yourself become completely sedentary. Therefore, an important strategy to avoid injury is keep yourself in reasonable condition throughout the year.

38. What is energy system training?

Modern-day sport training explains why a marathon runner is not trained to sprint from first to second base. The marathoners use their aerobic system in slow-twitch muscle fibers to run for several hours. It's only 90 feet between first and second base, but it's all anaerobic metabolism in fast-twitch fibers. Men and women all over the country prepare for the annual softball season by jogging, the exact opposite training for the sport of softball. The key to preparedness is to train the energy system you intend to use in competition.

The Energy Systems

A common belief with regard to energy for exercise is that oxygen combines with fuels such as carbohydrate and fat to produce energy. This is called aerobic metabolism and is the primary way we utilize food to produce the energy we use throughout the day. Aerobic exercise challenge our heart, lungs, and vascular system to provide blood and oxygen to working muscles. Aerobic exercise is usually presented as healthy exercise and is the only exercise that burns fat.

But sprinting does not use the aerobic system; oxygen is not involved at all. We have other ways of delivering energy without oxygen to provide quick energy. Aerobic activity takes time to begin since oxygen from the environment must be inhaled into the lung, delivered to the heart, and then delivered through the arteries to working muscles. The sprinter doesn't have time for all of this to happen; energy is needed immediately. Three ways of producing energy in the body are generally recognized. These are called energy systems.

ATP-PC System

All muscles contain a small supply of phosphagen substrates called ATP and PC. These phosphagens can be broken down immediately to provide instant energy. No oxygen is required. Although this system is wonderfully simple and immediate, there is only enough ATP-PC in the muscle for about 6–8 seconds of high-intensity exercise. It is the predominant energy system we use for high-speed activities like sprinting a 50-yard dash or throwing a shot put.

Lactic Acid System

Meanwhile, the second system can provide energy but is slightly slower. The carbohydrate stored in muscle is metabolized quickly, without oxygen. This takes about 10 chemical reactions with the final reaction producing lactic acid. Lactic acid is the product. This system starts to kick in around 8 seconds and reaches its limit after about 90 seconds. The advantage of this system is that it provides quick energy, but the disadvantage is that lactic acid is produced, decreasing the pH of the working muscles and causing fatigue. The lactic acid energy system is often called the intermediate system as it operates until the slower aerobic system is fully operational.

Aerobic Energy System

The aerobic system is a great system; it just takes some time to get started. Once operating, no problematic by-products are made except carbon dioxide and water. Oxygen combines with both carbohydrate and fat to produce almost unlimited energy. How fast oxygen can be delivered to the muscles, generally quantified as VO_{2max}, determines the power of the aerobic system.

The ATP-PC and lactic acid are two anaerobic energy systems. These three energy systems do not turn on and off but operate all the time. As a result, each may contribute more or less to various exercises, primarily determined by the time in which one is engaged. Table 5 suggests how these systems overlap.

Careful observation of the table leads one to the conclusion that most sport activities involve multiple energy systems. There are no hard rules for the exact percentage necessary in any one game, especially since the style of play and the position on the field or court is different. But with few exceptions, playing competitive sports requires one to train in all three energy systems. If you just observe one soccer player during a game, you will notice periods of walking, jogging, sprinting a short distance, and sprinting for longer distances. All energy systems are involved. A simple jogging program will not prepare one for soccer or any other ball game. If one ignores one of the energy systems and then needs it during

Table 5 Overlapping Energy Systems: Dependent on Time and Intensity

Zone	Performance Time	Major Energy System	Examples
Short bursts of high energy	0–6 seconds	ATP-PC	Shot put 40-meter dash Volleyball spike
High-energy activity at slightly slower pace	6–30 seconds	ATP and lactic acid	200-meter dash 25-meter freestyle Soccer play
Slightly reduced speed	2–3 minutes	Lactic acid and aerobic	800-meter run Second half of 1,500-meter run
Steady-paced activity	>3 minutes	Aerobic	Long run or bike ride Hiking

competition, they place themselves at risk. Training for high-level sport competition is complicated since most require a combination of all three energy systems.

Table 6 presents some suggested contributions for various activities and sports.

Energy Systems—How to Train

Early research in the 1950s indicated that individuals could perform significantly higher quality training when exercising in intervals than continuously. Interval training is composed of a combination of exercise intervals coupled with recovery intervals. Interval training is the predominant method to train energy systems. Table 7 presents an example of a simplified version of specific interval training.

Many people train their aerobic systems by performing continuous training. However, high-quality aerobic training usually involves some sort of interval training. Numerous variations of interval training have been designed, but the time of performance is the variable that changes little. To primarily use the ATP-PC system, you have to train at very high intensities but briefly. If the exercise is not brief, then you begin using more of the lactic acid system. You must also rest between intervals, allowing recovery so you can repeat high-intensity work. The lactic acid system is not primarily challenged unless the exercise lasts more than 15 seconds, so intervals need to be at least that long. Training the lactic acid system often involves incomplete recovery.

Table 6 Proposed Energy System Requirements for Selected Activities

Activity	ATP-PC	Lactic Acid	Aerobic
Volleyball	H	L	M
Soccer goalie	H	L	L
Soccer midfielder	H	H	M
Field hockey	H	H	M
Football receiver	H	M	M
Football lineman	H	M	L
Squash	H	H	M
10,000-meter run	L	L	H
1,500-meter swim	L	L	H

Table 7 Suggested Training Examples for Energy System Training

System	Activity	Rest	Rest Activity
ATP-PC	Run 10 40-yard dashes	60 seconds	Rest
Lactic acid	Run 9 200-yard dashes	60 seconds	Walk or light jog
Aerobic	Run 800 meters	90 seconds	Walk
	Swim 200 meters		Swim slowly

Interval training, especially lactic acid training, is tough. Athletes need to be well motivated to complete a difficult lactic acid workout. Muscles are very fatigued, and there is discomfort. Consequently, lactic acid training should not occur every day and such training should be interspersed with milder training. It takes about 60 minutes for lactic acid to be removed, so it is not wise to use such training at the beginning of a longer training session. Contrary to what some people believe, lactic acid is not around the day after training and cannot be removed by stretching or warm-up. Following a tough lactic acid training session, the athlete should perform mild aerobic exercise like slow jogging or walking for 15–20 minutes to help remove lactic acid.

Muscle Fiber Recruitment

Running a marathon uses the same leg muscles as you might use for sprinting, but the specific muscle fibers within the muscle are different. Human muscles are composed of slow-twitch (ST) and fast-twitch (FT)

fibers. ST fibers are smaller, have very good blood supply, and are primarily used during aerobic activities. Most activities done throughout the day use ST fibers almost exclusively. FT fibers are bigger, faster, stronger, but do not have much endurance. All muscles are composed of a combination of ST and FT fibers. The specific fibers are recruited for explicit activities. Longer slower activities use ST fibers while higher intensity activities use FT.

The Importance of Specificity

Specificity, the most important principle in exercise training, simply explains the preceding two sections. The body adapts specifically to the demands of training. The best training to achieve high performance and injury reduction is to specifically adapt to those activities one will use during competition. Jogging is a great activity for general aerobic fitness and to prepare for a road race, but competitive sports do not involve jogging. Training for competitive sports usually involves high-intensity training, replicating the exact activities that would be required when the game begins. Training in this manner, training the right energy system and recruiting the exact muscles to be used in competition, is the way to perform better and avoid injury.

39. How do you train to prevent overuse injuries while also improving performance?

Overuse injuries are subtle injuries, creeping up on one without a single, identifiable traumatic cause. Pain is felt in the knee, shoulder, or calf, but the participant does not remember any particular event that caused the pain. Excessive loading, insufficient recovery, and under preparedness cause overuse injuries. Athletes and nonathletes are susceptible. All parts of the musculoskeletal system can suffer overuse, but the muscle/tendon unit and bones are the primary targets. Acute injuries, like ligament and muscle tears, receive most of the attention in the lay media, but overuse injuries account for much of the time loss for athletes.

Fitness literature is ripe with all the ways to get fit. There is no dearth of suggestions on how to get fit, which equipment to buy, and video programming by people who seem to do nothing but work out. Rest and recovery are rarely mentioned; there's no money or excitement in resting. Earlier, athletes used to play sports seasonally, but athletes now tend to specialize, playing one sport all year. Coaches do not want their athletes to spend time away from the team. There is tremendous pressure to train 12 months a year.

Training errors cause overuse injuries. As previously discussed, training results in adaptation. Training stresses the body; during the recovery period, the musculoskeletal tissues that were stressed recover and get stronger. If training and heavy loading continue without recovery, the healing process is overwhelmed; maladaptation occurs. Tendons and bones tend to lose their structure and weaken. Localized pain occurs when exercising and appears without any memory of injury. If therapy is not applied at this point, athletes often will not be able to continue a season of play.

The best procedure is to avoid overuse injuries in the first place. Training involves repetition; whether it is running distances or hitting forehands in tennis, repetitions are necessary for skill acquisition. Repeated practicing brings about change, but excessive repetitions are the cause of overuse injury. Athletes want to practice, but if they practice too hard they get hurt. Fortunately, there are strategies one can use to practice and achieve while avoiding overuse.

Fatigue and Overuse

As discussed in Question 41, when muscles contract they help stabilize joints. But what happens when muscles are fatigued? The answer comes from research conducted at the University of Waterloo in Ontario. Researchers took x-ray images of subjects as they moved their arms through different positions. They were interested in how much the head of the humerus moved when the arm moved. After taking careful measurements of the head of the humerus, they put the subjects through a fatiguing protocol of the shoulder muscles. Subsequent x-ray measurements indicated considerable drift of the head of the humerus. The muscles stabilizing the shoulder were too fatigued to hold the shoulder in place, consequently putting considerable strain on the shoulder capsule as well as the tendon/muscle connection. When muscles are fatigued, they cannot stabilize the joint, and additional stress is placed on those tendons surrounding the joints. This strain on tendons is one cause of overuse.

Fatigue is also related to the overall stress. Little League baseball teams in southern California often play baseball all year. Age group swim teams often practice year round. Young athletes often play on multiple teams in the same season, playing on a school team and a club team at the same time. Studies show that when athletes have less than two rest days a week they are 5.2 times more likely to experience an overuse injury. Athletes need rest not only during the actual practice but also during the week and during the year.

How to Create Practice Drills without Joint Fatigue

Skill acquisition requires repetition. Players need to hit many shots in order to gain precision. One strategy is to create practice to bring about change without excessive joint fatigue. Fortunately, research in Motor Learning helps with this problem.

Massed versus Distributed Learning

There are two basic ways of presenting practice drills. Let's say you want athletes to hit 50 forehand drives in tennis. They can either hit 50 drives in a row (massed practice) or 10 shots in a row 5 separate times (distributed). In each case, they will hit 50 forehand drives. Distributed practice is better at improving retention; the ability to perform later is improved more when practice is distributed. In terms of reducing injury, distributed practice allows recovery, less fatigue of shoulder muscles, and less overuse. Distributed practice helps more with performance and decreases the muscular fatigue related to injury.

Contextual Interference

A second series of motor learning studies relates to what researchers call contextual interference. Sounds complicated, but this is just related to mixing things up. Let's use the tennis example again. Think of going out onto the tennis court and setting up a ball machine to throw the ball 20 times in a row to your forehand. Now go back and have the machine throw 20 balls but mix them up so that you don't know where the ball is going to go; that is contextual interference. Like distributed practice, mixing it up results in better retention. That is, mixing up shots makes a better player, and since you are not doing the exact movement each time, there is less fatigue, less overuse.

A final question regarding practice is whether highly repetitious drills actually make better performers. The principle of specificity suggests otherwise. Practice should replicate play. For example, baseball pitchers are often asked to throw multiple high-speed pitches in a row during practice, even though most pitchers throw less than 15 pitches in an inning, most interspersed with rest. It is possible to achieve great success in sports that require extensive accuracy and practice; the key is not to overly fatigue joint muscles.

Kinetic Chain and Overuse Injury

Nolan Ryan was an All Star baseball pitcher, pitching for 27 years. Amazingly successful, he routinely threw the ball over 100 mph; he was remarkably healthy. One reason for his success was his beautiful motion—the kinetic chain. The kinetic chain is a natural form of movement leading to throwing, striking, or kicking. The kinetic chain is the transfer of momentum from the ground through the leg, hip, trunk, shoulder, elbow, wrist, and hand. As force is transmitted through the body, the individual stress on any one part is reduced. On the other hand, a broken chain results in one vulnerable part of the body (like the elbow) receiving too much strain. Ryan's chain was so perfect he did not experience such strain. The kinetic chain is seen in many sports including golf, tennis, and many field events in athletics.

Many times when one is learning a sport, little time is spent trying to perfect the kinetic chain. Often, considerable attention is placed on developing accuracy. But too much attention to accuracy often results in poor mechanics. Studies have shown that velocity training is more important than accuracy training when developing the kinetic chain. The natural tendency to transfer force through the body, through the kinetic chain, occurs more readily when trying to swing, hit, or throw harder. But as soon as a target is put up, novices will reduce their natural movements in order to hit a target. Developing the kinetic chain is of paramount importance when learning a new sport and requires professional instruction.

Stress Fractures

Running sports are the primary activities that result in stress fractures to the lower body. Cross-country and track athletes are particularly susceptible, as well as field athletes such as soccer players. Women are more susceptible than men. You cannot train through a stress fracture; it will only get worse, so the best thing to do is get treatment immediately upon experiencing localized pain. The treatment normally consists of a reduction in training. Athletes do not want to stop training, but athletes need to be convinced that continued training makes the injury worse, possibly leading to a complete break in the bone.

Several risk factors are prevalent, including training on hard surfaces, training in shoes older than six months, and always running on a track in the same direction. Females who have menstrual dysfunction, poor nutrition, and less bone density are at greater risk. One risk factor is unpreparedness. That is, athletes start practice without preparation, increasing intensity and volume too quickly to adapt. This is also true for another overuse injury of the lower body—medial tibial stress syndrome. Stress fractures are clearly an overuse injury and are caused by excessive training without sufficient recovery. Here are some suggestions to avoid stress fractures.

1. Get in shape prior to the competitive season. Use strength training to strengthen leg muscles. Slowly increase mileage and back off if you feel any localized pain.
2. Build rest days into each week of training. Mild workouts should follow tough workouts.
3. Specialize your training. That is, don't jump rope or do a lot of stair running if you're playing soccer or running track.
4. For females with menstrual dysfunction, see your physician to obtain advice on maintaining a eumenorrheic cycle.
5. Maintain a healthy diet.
6. Avoid running on hard surfaces, especially those that slope, causing extra stress unilaterally.
7. Make sure you have proper footwear. Try to buy footwear from a shoe store that has trained personnel.
8. If localized pain repeats during the latter stages of exercise, see a qualified medical professional for help.

40. What is overtraining syndrome, and how can I prevent it?

In 1996, prior to the Olympic Games in Atlanta, the first International Conference on Overtraining was held. Until this time, coaches and athletes around the world were aware of periods in many athletes' careers when performance diminished, even when they were training hard. Athletes became listless, bored, burned out. Two conditions were identified at this important conference:

- Overreaching: An accumulation of training and nontraining stress resulting in a short-term decrement in performance—recovery usually takes a matter of days
- Overtraining: Long-term decrement in performance—athletes cannot be positively influenced by short rest—requires lengthy recovery

Overreaching is relatively common, most often occurring at the beginning of a competitive season. Athletes start a preseason, often in poor condition, and train very strenuously. Instead of getting better, there is a decrement in performance. A few days of reduced intensity or rest allows the athlete to recover. But overtraining is much more serious, and recovery can actually take months. Overtraining is a relatively new phenomenon, occurring more often in the past 30 years. It was this recognition that prompted the 1996 conference.

Professional athletes are particularly susceptible. But overtraining is not exclusive to professional athletes as college and even some high school athletes are susceptible. Anyone who trains vigorously throughout the year, especially if the training routine doesn't change, is at risk of overtraining.

Like overuse injuries, overtraining is an imbalance between training and recovery. But the stressors on an individual are more than just exercise training. For example, athletes in school are constantly balancing the stress of high-intensity training, competition, studying, exams, financial concerns, and social conflict. All of these combine to place considerable 24-hour stress on an athlete. It doesn't take that much for the athlete to become overwhelmed.

There are a number of causes of overtraining, including:

- Too much overall stress and pressure
- Too much practice and physical training
- Physical exhaustion and allover soreness
- Boredom because of too much repetition
- Underrecovery

The most common symptom of overtraining is a decrement in performance. Regardless of how hard an athlete may be training, they are less successful. Typical symptoms are as follows:

- Decreased immune response—athletes are more prone to infection and illness
- Decreased performance
- Quitting/burnout
- Increased risk of injury—especially overuse injuries

Preventing Overtraining

Periodization is one strategy to prevent overtraining. The basic tenets of periodization are as follows:

- Athletes cannot stay in top condition all year.
- Intense periods of training and competition must be followed by periods of reduced activity—recovery.
- Periodized training involves planned recovery.
- An annual plan to peak and then rest is required.
- Planned recovery is required.

Table 8 Four Month Periodized Training Model

Months	1	1	1	1	1
Competitions	None	None	Minor	Main	None
Periods	Preparatory	Increased Preparatory	Precompetitive	Competition	Rest

Periodization requires an annual plan, a plan that results in specific periods during the year when an athlete peaks followed by recovery. Athletes might go through two or three periods a year, but each is followed by recovery. A cycle might look like this four-month cycle given in table 8.

A major benefit of periodization is that athletes plan to engage in peak competition for only a few weeks and then recover. Periodization requires planning. Each week is planned, as well as the entire cycle. Each cycle starts with relatively high volume, allowing the body to strengthen and adapt. During the early part of the cycle, intensity is low. As the cycle progresses, volume is reduced as intensity is increased. If volume is not reduced, then the athlete will start to experience overuse injury.

Periodization was originally planned exclusively for strength and power athletes, but this model can be used for any activity in which an individual intends to compete. Road racers can use this model, planning for the big 5K event. Tournament players in tennis, squash, and badminton can create their own periodized plan, starting each cycle with renewed vigor.

Fitness participants can also use the basic principles of periodization to improve their training. One of the biggest causes of overtraining, besides the absence of rest, is boredom. Repeating the same workout day in and day out year after year results in staleness and burnout. Workouts need to be changed periodically throughout the year, possibly starting a new cycle every three months or so. Using the seasons is a good way to change one's routines. Fitness is maintained, and overtraining is prevented. A true periodized model is probably not required for most fitness participants, but here are some recommendations that will avoid burnout, overtraining, and overuse.

1. Remember that you cannot be in top shape all year. Allow for periodic reductions in training.
2. Mix up training methods throughout the year. Create novel training. Try a new activity.
3. When exercise begins to feel like a job, change the activity.
4. Find activities that result in fun. Play is the verb for sport. We **play** sports.

41. What's the best way to strength train, and how will this help prevent injury?

Strength training has been around since the ancient Greek Olympics, but the benefits of strength training have risen and fallen over time. Controversial statements such as "strength training will stunt your growth," "weight lifting will make you muscle bound, reducing your ability to move," and "strength training will make you slower" have confounded participants. Although none of these statements is true, common beliefs are hard to dispel. Most people now believe in the benefits of strength (resistance) training. Coaches and trainers recommend strength training for athletes, and pediatricians recommend strength training for youth. Seniors participate in resistance training with very positive results.

While aerobic training improves the ability to endure, resistance training improves our ability to lift or move things, to maintain posture, to do tasks that require short-term effort. Daily tasks such as cleaning house, gardening, and many recreational activities require strength. Being stronger gives us better balance and agility, helps prevent falling, and allows us to participate in activities that require strength. With regard to injury, strong muscles resist injury.

In Question 39, the example of what happens to the stability of the shoulder when shoulder muscles are fatigued is described. When muscles contract, they tend to move bones in a prescribed manner, but each muscle contraction also has a stabilizing component, a force that holds the joint together. This is evident in rehabilitation programs in which resistance training is a critical part of rehabilitation. Resistance training restores stability.

The amount of strength training varies by need. Athletes involved in power sports like shot putting and discus throwing need tremendous strength. Athletes involved in contact sports like football, ice hockey, and lacrosse need strength. Virtually all athletes need some form of strength training to perform and reduce injury. Strength training programs are recommended for the general public, but often not as intense.

Modern-day strength training started after World War II, when so many soldiers returned home and needed rehabilitation. DeLorme and Watkins used various reps, sets, and RMs to describe their program. A rep is one repetition of an exercise, while a set is a group of reps one does without rest. An RM is considered a repetition maximum. For example, a 10 RM is a weight one can lift 10 times but fails on rep number 11. Researchers have conducted literally hundreds of studies using various combinations to increase strength.

Although you may not think so when reviewing the plethora of strength training books, resistance training is not that complicated. Lifting free weights like barbells and dumbbells has been the standard resistance training method. But companies have built elaborate machines designed to stabilize the body while performing strength exercises. Many people now use kettlebells, elastic bands, and body resistance exercises like push-ups, pull-ups, and squats. Regardless of methodology, people will get stronger if they repeatedly lift a heavy weight, a weight that cannot be moved more than 10–20 times, on a regular basis.

The American College of Sports Medicine recommends two days of some form of resistance training each week. Competitive athletes will normally train much harder, especially those in power sports. The primary difference between programs for competitive athletes and programs for the general population is intensity. The average participant can achieve their recommendation by performing one set of 6–8 exercises twice a week. The resistance should be intense enough, where the exercise is progressively difficult and fatiguing in the end. Exercising to failure is not required. Enthusiasts may perform two to three sets of the same exercises, resulting in slightly better results.

Which Exercises Should You Use?

When you go into most fitness gyms, you are faced with a huge array of resistance equipment (usually called VRMs). For novices, the view is daunting. Don't try all of the machines. Find just a few exercises that train the basic body parts. Use exercises that are slightly more complex, exercises that are multijoint. Doing things like arm curls or triceps extensions are unnecessary, as you can exercise these same body parts with multijoint exercises. You are also striving for symmetry, training all the body. The following chart in table 9 presents four basic multijoint exercises that train the basic body parts.

Doing any of these exercises with regularity will make you stronger. Variable resistance machines (VRMs) are fairly easy to use; increasing or decreasing the resistance is just a matter of moving a pin. VRMs are a good way to start, but once you have developed some confidence with resistance training, try some free weight or body weight exercises. An advantage of VRMs is expedience, but a disadvantage is that you do not have to stabilize your body. Free weight and body weight exercises require you to stabilize your body, an important contribution to this form of strength training.

Table 9 Suggested Resistance Exercises using Variable Resistance Machines, Free Weights, or Body Weight

Body Area	Variable Resistance Machine*	Free Weights	Body Weight
Chest	Chest press machine	Bench press	Push-ups
Upper back	Rowing machine	Bent over rows	Inverted pull-ups
Latissimus and lower back	Lat pull-down machine	Pull overs on bench	Pull-ups
Thigh	Leg press machine	Squats with weight	Free squats

Variable resistance machines (VRM) are the standard fixed motion exercise machines in fitness gyms.

Strength Training for Sport

Strength training for sport requires intense effort. To gain strength, the resistance should be high. You should not be able to perform a high number of repetitions. Multiple sets of each exercise are required. Athletes need strength, but they also need to apply strength gained from the weight room to the playing field. Balance, coordination, and the kinetic chain are important. Lifting free weights develops not only strength but also balance and coordination. Lifting a free weight requires synchronous effort. For example, the clean is one of the basic free weight exercises. There are several ways of performing a clean, but all require coordination and a transfer of momentum from one phase to another. The clean helps develop the kinetic chain. Performing front squats requires the athlete to balance the weight. Not only is leg strength developed, but the muscles of the trunk are also involved. Athletes will also benefit from body weight exercises as well as exercises with dumbbells and kettlebells.

Periodized Strength Training

Periodized strength training is very effective, involving a systematic manipulation of volume and intensity leading to peak strength and power. Studies show that periodized strength results in greater gains than traditional linear programs.

There are many models for periodized strength training. Following planned rest, the athlete starts over, albeit stronger. Table 10 describes one.

Table 10 Periodized Strength Training Model

Goal of Period	Hypertrophy	Strength	Power	Peaking	Rest
Weeks	4	3	3	2	1
Sets/exercise	3–5	3–5	3–5	13–	
Reps	8–12	4–8	2–4	1–3	
Intensity	Low	Moderate	High	Very high	
Volume	Very high	High	Moderate	Low	

From the Weight Room to the Playing Field

Strength gained in the weight room must be applied to be effective. Weight room exercises should be functional to the needs of the sport involved. Training with a purpose is one key to functional strength. For example, with few exceptions most sports are played in a standing position. Therefore, most strength exercises should be done in a standing position. Don't waste time performing exercises that have no benefit. For example, with few exceptions athletic movements require multiple joints. Performing single joint exercises like arm curls is not functional.

One may be strong but not powerful. Powerful athletes can exert significant force quickly. There is no question that strength training improves power, but additional power training supports the transfer of strength gained in the weight room to power for use on the playing field. Typical power training activities include:

- High-speed sprints—short sprints
- Hill running—running full speed up the hill for about 6–8 seconds
- Stair running—running full speed up stairs for about 6–8 seconds
- Medicine ball throws—throwing medicine balls for maximum distance
- Plyometric exercises

Plyometric Exercises

Plyometric exercises are designed to enhance the stretch-shortening cycle of the muscle/tendon unit. Rapidly stretching a muscle/tendon unit enhances the subsequent muscle contraction. Athletes naturally use this stretch-shortening cycle (SSC) to jump higher or throw farther. Just observe an athlete performing a vertical jump; you will notice a rapid three-joint flexion of the hip, knee, and ankle just prior to jumping. The rapid flexion stretches the joint tendons resulting in a higher jump. Plyometric training facilitates the SSC.

Plyometric training is stressful on muscles and tendons, and athletes must start slowly with this form of training. Start first with various forms of hopping, repeated jumping, and one-legged hopping. Once the athlete is comfortable with low-level training, they can start with depth jumping. Depth jumping places additional stress on the lengthening tendons, improving the SSC. If an athlete stands on a bench that is 12 inches high and jumps off, the resultant stretch on the hip, knee, and ankle tendons is enhanced. Depth jumping involves jumping off a platform or bench that is 6–30 inches high followed immediately by a maximum jump. The goal is to jump as high and quickly as possible. Multiple depth jumping is to jump up and down over a series of 6–10 benches as quickly as possible. Bench height should be reduced if athletes tend to lose leg stability. Many fitness gyms have Plyo boxes, but these are often used incorrectly. For example, participants are simply encouraged to jump as high as possible onto a box. This is not depth jumping or plyometrics.

Year-Round Training

Strength training should be year-round, training interspersed with rest. Training should involve ebb and flow, a time to gain strength and a time to rest. Participants should develop multiple routines, changing them throughout the year. Fortunately, strength gains are not lost quickly, so time off does not hurt; it helps. Power training should not be conducted all year. The best practice is to create a power training program to peak when the competitive season begins. Regardless of your strength training protocol, sound functional strength results in better athletes who are more resistant to injury.

42. How flexible do I need to be? Should I do a lot of stretching before I play?

Why do people spend so much time working on their flexibility? Is there some reason why we might profit from an extensive range of motion? Flexibility is generally defined as one's range of motion (ROM). Yes, we need to be able to tie our shoes, put on our clothes without restriction, and reach overhead to wash our hair. But do we need extreme ROM? Is extreme ROM good for us? With regard to flexibility, injury, and performance there are four basic questions:

- Does static stretching prior to performance reduce injury rate?
- Does static stretching prior to performance improve performance?
- Do flexible people have fewer injuries? Perform better?
- Should we have flexibility training in our fitness program?

Static stretching prior to athletic performance has been routine, as the general belief was that stretching prior to performance allowed muscles to contract more easily, reducing muscle/tendon injury. The efficacy of static stretching prior to performance has received little research support. In fact, some studies have even shown that static stretching has a negative effect on subsequent high-speed or power events. One problem with static stretching was when athletes substituted static stretching for warm-up. Real warm-up may have been reduced. Warm-up reduces the rate of injury. Static stretching does not increase the temperature of the working muscle.

The majority of studies have shown that pre-event stretching does not reduce injury rate. There may be some mild positive effect on muscle/tendon strain, but that remains very tenuous. Meanwhile, stretching is ingrained into many people's beliefs, and many prefer to perform some stretching exercises prior to performance. So if someone wants to go through a static stretching routine prior to performance, it doesn't seem contraindicated. If this makes one comfortable, there seems no ill effect.

With regard to pre-event stretching and performance, there is no research in support of including pre-event stretching, especially static stretching. Many athletes, especially in track and field, will use some form of dynamic stretching prior to performance. This involves swinging legs and arms through an extended ROM. Since sport is dynamic, dynamic stretching seems more appropriate to prepare an athlete for movement. Some dynamic warm-ups even mimic the subsequent activity. Unfortunately, available research has not confirmed that dynamic warm-up assists performance.

Researchers at Louisiana State University have found that statically stretching muscles just prior to activities that involve speed and power reduced performance. For example, sprinting speed was reduced following static stretching. Reduction in power and speed is most detrimental right after stretching, especially if the stretching is longer in duration. Although many athletes prefer some form of static stretching prior to performance, immediate pre-performance stretching is contraindicated.

Flexibility, Injury, and Performance

Some people are naturally more flexible than others. For example, some people have joint laxity that may actually contribute to injury. A joint that is too loose is not stable. A loose shoulder joint tends to sublux (the humerus moves out and back in the socket) when stressed. Loose knees and ankles are particularly problematic. So extensive flexibility is not generally positive in the prevention of injury.

Since injuries happen during the normal ROM, one must question why an athlete needs more flexibility than required. Athletes only need sufficient ROM to successfully perform their sport. Every sport activity has an individual requirement. Hurdlers have to have very flexible hips, lower backs, and hamstrings. Gymnasts and divers need widespread flexibility. Swimmers and tennis players need flexible shoulders. The activity of the sport naturally provides the stress to maintain and develop the ROM required. Excessive supplementary exercises are unnecessary.

Range of Motion and Rehabilitation

One of the immediate effects of an injury is a reduction in ROM. Bleeding and damage to soft tissues tends to reduce motion. Following surgery, joints are very stiff, often having been in a cast or sling for weeks. Regaining ROM is one of the basic treatments during rehabilitation. Regaining motion is best done by moving slowly through the ROM. Therapists will often manually move affected joints. Heat is often used prior to treatment in order to facilitate movement. Regaining ROM is often difficult, but a gradual regaining of ROM is in order. Individuals are not normally ready to return to full competition until normalcy has returned.

Flexibility Training in the Fitness Routine

Only a few generations ago, daily physical activity was normal for most people. Modern-day innovation has changed the physical requirement for day-to-day life. Meanwhile, our bodies are the same—have the same requirements. People tend to sit more than ever, often bent over their computer screen in their workstation. Further, many do not have a high-quality ergonomic workstation. The result of this constant sitting is reduced flexibility of the hamstrings, lower back, and upper back. Many flex their necks too much during the day and rarely put their hands over their heads.

As a result, ROM decreases. Further, as an individual ages, joints become stiffer because of age and inactivity. Some flexibility training is in order. Dynamic and static stretching both work. Dynamic stretching works better prior to a workout while static stretching is easier to do at the end of a workout, when the body is warm. Stretches longer than 30 seconds are unnecessary. Typical body segments are neck and shoulder, lower back, hamstring, and calf. One only needs to do a few exercises two to three times a week.

43. How can I minimize the chance of getting a concussion?

As discussed in Question 28, a single concussion is a mild brain injury, but subsequent or multiple concussions present serious problems. Many sports medicine professionals believe that one basic key to concussion prevention is education. For example, studies have shown that many athletes are still not aware of the symptoms of concussion presented in Question 28. In such cases, athletes may continue playing, risking a serious second impact. Many schools do not have a certified athletic trainer, and concussion protocols are left to the coach. And many concussions occur during practice when athletic trainers are not in attendance. In such cases, the coach is in charge when injuries occur. Anyone who has received a significant blow to the head needs to stop play and obtain medical support.

Unfortunately, coaches may either ignore or are unaware of protocol. It is not unusual for a coach to have never taken a course in sports medicine, yet they are in control when injuries occur. The absence of any formal education is particularly true in youth sport where volunteers do most of the coaching.

Football is the primary sport causing concussions, but participants in ice hockey, soccer, and basketball are frequently affected. As a result, many high school and college programs, as well as youth programs, have instituted concussion protocols. Many schools have reduced and even eliminated contact during football practice sessions. Organized sports are not the only group to address concussions, as helmet wearing during bicycling is now almost universal. Many downhill skiers now wear helmets. All of these efforts have paid off, as people are now more aware of the hazards of concussions.

The following are some basic recommendations for reducing concussions.

Wear the Appropriate Helmet

Many sports have a mandated helmet requirement. When there is a set standard, the helmet should be certified by the National Operating Committee on Standards for Athletic Equipment (NOCSAE). Considerable research is in process on helmet design. Progress has been made, but no helmet is "concussion proof." Helmets are specific to different sports, so wear the appropriate helmet. The helmet must fit as studies have shown that most football helmets do not fit properly. In addition, all players should have the same quality helmet. Second-string players should not have inferior equipment. The helmet, with chin strap, should be worn in practice, not just during games.

Educate Players

A major concern in sports medicine is that the helmet actually supports the athlete's belief of invincibility. Players must be taught that aggressive play does not mean leading with the head. Players in football must be taught to block and tackle appropriately without leading by the head. Coaches must support the officials to eliminate unfair play. Players must be able to communicate with coaches and trainers without punitive measures or ridicule. Players must be aware of the consequences of concussion and appreciate the fact that all players are susceptible regardless of skill and attitude. Any athlete who has received a hit to the head should be stopped and evaluated regardless of the situation.

Neck Muscles, Mouthpieces, and Shields

Studies have shown that athletes with stronger neck muscles tend to absorb force better, thereby reducing the risk of concussion. Female athletes tend to have weaker neck muscles, so strengthening neck muscles is in order. Some studies have suggested that mouthpieces may attenuate shock on the brain, thereby reducing concussion severity. There is no conclusive evidence of this, but a mouthpiece is a good idea most of the time. Face shields are worn in some ice hockey leagues. Some research suggests that a face shield may reduce concussion severity. Face shields also reduce other facial injuries, so they should be worn in games and practices.

People involved in sport are going to receive concussions. But behavior and education can reduce the incidence. Considering the possible negative long-term effects of concussion, everyone needs to understand the consequence. Doing the right thing is not bravery; it is smart.

44. How do I reduce the frequency of shoulder and elbow injuries?

The shoulder, elbow, wrist, and fingers are the last link in the kinetic chain that moves from the ground, through the body. As discussed in

Question 39, the kinetic chain takes considerable stress off individual joints. One of the most important ways to reduce shoulder and elbow injuries is to develop this chain. All parts of the body are connected, so when one segment of the chain is injured, subsequent parts of the body receive more stress. Form is of critical importance when preventing any injury; the shoulder and elbow are particularly sensitive to errors in form.

When we think of the shoulder joint, we often think of the humerus moving in its socket on the scapula (shoulder blade). But the shoulder is much more complex, as the wide range of movements of the shoulder also involve movements of the scapula. Such freedom of movement comes with greater need for stability by muscles and tendons surrounding the joint. In general, there are three sets of muscles affecting the shoulder: the large muscles that move the scapula, the large muscles that move the humerus, and the rotator cuff muscles.

Injuries to the shoulder are caused by falling, acute stress, and overuse. Falling is the chief cause of a shoulder separation, a tear of the ligament that holds the scapula and clavicle (collar bone) together. Dislocations can also occur when falling, primarily when one puts their arm out to stop the fall. The best way to reduce falling injuries is to learn how to fall. Martial arts participants and gymnasts are great at falling as they simply tuck their head and shoulder and roll without injury. Athletes in many sports, including mountain biking, should practice performing a shoulder roll to prevent this injury. Overuse is mostly related to throwing.

One of the most important motor skills is the overhand throwing motion. This motion is evident in activities like the tennis serve, badminton overhead, volleyball spike and serve, and javelin throw. Developing good mechanics through the kinetic chain is one of the most important developmental activities for anyone involved in overhand activity. Besides learning to fall and developing the kinetic chain, several training practices can reduce overuse shoulder injury.

Train to Reduce Shoulder Injury

1. Maintain strong shoulder muscles. Some years back, strength exercises for throwers were contraindicated as athletes were led to believe that the range of motion would decrease. But if resistance exercises require mobility and flexibility exercises are also utilized, range of motion is not compromised. Strengthening the shoulder muscles, including those muscles of the scapula, the big muscles of the shoulder, and the rotator cuff, is a good start. If any of these areas is weak, the kinetic chain is weak.

Resistance exercises for the shoulder should include a balance of pushing and pulling exercises. For example, pushing activities involve muscles in front of the shoulder while pulling strengthens upper back muscles. Overhead movement as well as rotation of the humerus should also be involved. Resistance exercise should involve the complete range of motion using a combination of barbell, dumbbell, and kettlebell weights. Rotator cuff muscles require a bit more specificity. Rotator cuff exercises are gentler exercises, not explosive. Form is important. Internal and external rotations are both important functions of the rotator cuff. A good resource (listed in the "Directory of Resources") is the Throwers Ten. This is a list of 10 exercises designed to strengthen those muscles utilized in throwing, including the rotator cuff.

2. Maintain flexibility of the shoulder. As discussed in Question 42, extensive flexibility is not recommended, but one needs enough flexibility to smoothly go through the throwing motion. Throwing freely, without a target, will develop flexibility. Following a good warm-up, simply throw a ball against a wall or perform some long throws. Proper stretching to keep the shoulders and pectoral muscles loose is also important. A good stretch is a door (or corner) stretch. Place both forearms along the frame of the door with elbows at shoulder height. Slowly bring the chest forward into the door until a stretch is felt across chest and shoulders. Thirty seconds is all that is required for this to work. A fairly thorough shoulder mobility routine is provided in the "Directory of Resources."

3. Since so many of the injuries to the shoulder are overuse injuries, practicing correctly, without overly fatiguing the shoulder muscles, is important. The acquisition of skill requires extensive practice, but too much practice without recovery results in an overuse injury. Question 39 discusses the procedure for how to practice without overusing.

4. The first thing to do before any practice is to warm up. Performing the exact skill involved in your sport is the warm-up procedure. Baseballers should throw overhand, and tennis players should serve. Start with easy throws or hits, slowly warming up the muscles until the movement is unencumbered.

5. Use a rest or easy day between hard practice sessions. Repeated hard days do not allow for recovery.

Preventing Elbow Injuries

Question 19 describes the anatomy and motion of the elbow joint. When throwing or striking an object like a tennis ball, movement occurs in the shoulder, elbow, and forearm. The two common sources of pain at the elbow are lateral epicondylitis (often called tennis elbow) and medial epicondylitis (golfer's elbow or baseball elbow). Pain on the outside of the elbow (lateral epicondylitis) most often occurs in racket sports, particularly the backhand. Pain on the inside of the elbow (medial epicondylitis) occurs in golfers, but much more often in baseball pitchers. Another elbow pain is bruising of the ulnar nerve, commonly caused by falling on one's elbow.

Almost all elbow pain is caused by overuse. It is possible to sprain the elbow, especially by putting the hand down when falling, so learning to fall is important. Overuse remains the big problem for the elbow, and such injuries can be reduced by the following guidelines:

1. Warm up prior to play. This is the rule for all athletic activities but even more important for shoulder and elbow. Use related warm-up to perform the exact activity expected during play, starting slowly and working toward higher intensity activity.
2. Since overuse is the biggest cause of elbow pain, every attempt must be made to train properly. The practice methods outlined in Question 39 are a good start. Baseball pitching is one of the primary causes of pain on the inside of the elbow. For years, the advice was to not allow youth to throw curve balls, but studies show that fastball pitching causes the most stress on the inside of the elbow. Too much high-speed throwing causes a significant increase in injury. Pitching every day should be avoided, and pitching all year should be avoided.
    Start slowly to give the arm time to adjust early in the season. This means fewer pitches in the early season, allowing the arm to adapt. Following a pitching workout, stretching the shoulder, elbow, and forearm is a good practice. If you are sore, ice might be a good therapy, but if you are sore every time you pitch, you are overdoing it.
3. Strengthen muscles around the elbow and forearm. Many of the strengthening exercises for the shoulder also strengthen the elbow. However, strengthening the forearm requires some more specific exercises. One easy way is to stand with your elbow touching your side. Use the Thrower's Ten two to three times a week listed in the "Directory of Resources."
4. Form, or lack of it, is one of the primary causes of elbow pain. This is particularly true for the backhand in tennis, as many novice players tend to lead with the elbow, placing extreme stress on the elbow joint. This is one of the principal causes of lateral epicondylitis. A

two-handed backhand may be one solution for those players who have trouble hitting a backhand otherwise. Equipment is also a problem. The grip of the tennis racket should not be too big, placing extra stress on the forearm. Have a tennis professional help you select the right size racket.

Finally, when we train to prevent an injury in any one part of the body, it is important to understand that all joints are connected to one another in a chain. As a result, maintaining the strength and flexibility of all of our body is important, not just the shoulder or elbow. The body is a big chain, each part dependent on the other for support and the transfer of force. Train the entire body to be strong and flexible. Mobility and balance are required. Posture is particularly important. Maintain a healthy back and core (Question 45), strong legs, and healthy feet.

45. How should I train for a healthy back and core, and how will this help prevent injury?

Low back pain is one of the primary reasons that individuals seek medical care and is one of the primary causes of absenteeism at work. Older people are more susceptible, but anyone can suffer low back pain, including athletes. Over the years, treatment options have varied considerably from complete rest to extensive stretching and various abdominal exercises. Rest is a poor option for low back pain, and many abdominal exercises actually exacerbate back pain. Recently, the work of Dr. Stuart McGill at the University of Waterloo, in Waterloo, Ontario, has enlightened practitioners about the importance of core stability.

Stabilizing the core means to stabilize the spine, a series of 33 interlocking vertebrae. Since so many mobile parts originate off the spine, such as the shoulder girdle, hip girdle, and head, stability of the spine is vital for back health as well as performance. One analogy some have used to describe spine stabilization is to observe a radio tower. You will see multiple guy wires running from the ground to the tower, keeping it upright. What is important is that the wires support the tower in multiple directions, as the tower could fall in any direction. Interestingly, for some reason, in the past decade or so there has been an obsession with abdominal exercises, many searching for what some call the "six pack." Imagine if the radio tower only had guy wires on the north side; this is analogous to only improving core stability in one direction. Core stability means 360° stability.

Core stability is related to muscle strength and stiffness all around the spine. The core needs stability not only because of our upright posture but also because the spine is in the middle of the kinetic chain. As one generates momentum from the ground, it must travel through the core. A weak core results in a poor chain, as well as an overloaded spine.

Core muscles must be not only strong and mobile but also stiff to transfer kinetic chain forces. McGill has recommended that isometric exercises are an easy way to enhance stiffness with little risk of injury.

The Big 3

McGill highly recommends three basic exercises (see the "Directory of Resources") designed to improve core stability.

1. Curl up: Lie on your back with one knee bent and the other straight. Place your hands under your lower back and slowly raise your head and shoulders off the mat. Try to hold the position for about 10 seconds and then rest. This is not a sit-up; do not come up off the mat. The goal is to lift the head and shoulders without movement in the lower back.

    The tendency for many is to try this as many times as possible, repeating the exercise many times. The basic recommendation is to think of this as doing reps and sets (Question 41). Start with a set of five reps, each with a rest of about 10 seconds. Rest for 30 seconds or so, then do a set of three reps, then do one. As you get stronger, increase the number of reps, not the duration of the reps.
2. The side plank: Lie on your side with your legs bent and upper body, supported on your elbow. Now raise your hips off the mat and hold for 10 seconds. Use the same model of repetitions as for the curl up. Now switch sides and repeat. As you get stronger, modify the plank by doing things like raising from the extended leg, or using the hand as a support. Numerous progressions exist for this important exercise.
3. Bird dog: Assume an all-four position with knees on the mat or ground, arms straight down. While trying to keep your back straight and in a neutral position, make a fist and raise your left arm horizontal to the ground while you raise your right leg horizontal to the ground. Use the same rep system as described for the curl up. It is important to maintain a straight back during this exercise. If you start to round your back, decrease the time of each repetition. Also, if you cannot do this exercise, try just lifting the leg alone and then the arm alone to get started. Try other progressions as you strengthen.

Mobility Training

The three exercises given earlier are great for stabilizing the spine and should be considered part of any well-rounded exercise program. In addition, maintaining and developing spinal mobility is important. One exercise that is highly recommended for mobility is the Cat-Camel (also called the Mad Cat), an exercise that is safe and should be performed prior to the Big 3. To do this, assume an all-four position on your hands and knees. Slowly arch your entire spine and hips into a rounded position (like a camel hump). At the end, you should be looking down. Now switch into the opposite position with head looking up (the cat position) and a slight stretch to the lower back. Hold each position several times.

Additional Strength Training

Besides the Big 3 exercises, most people involved in vigorous sports strengthen their back and core with additional activities. Many of the core muscles originate off the hips, so hip stabilization is also important. The gluteal muscles connect the hips to the leg, so muscles that activate the gluteals assist with core stabilization. One basic exercise for the gluteals is a hip raise or bridge. To do this, lie on your back with your legs bent; tighten your gluteal and raise your hips from the ground or mat. Keep squeezing your glutes for five seconds and then return. Repeat this several times.

Traditionally, one of the basic resistance exercises for the lower back, glutes, and legs has been the dead lift. The rationale for the dead lift is that it is sequential, mimicking the kinetic chain. The dead lift is a good exercise but only if performed properly. Excessive flexion and extension of the back creates significant torque on the vertebrae and can cause injury. Squats are also good exercises, either with a barbell or by holding a dumbbell. Squats should be done with a neutral spine, no flexing or extending. Deep squats while holding a dumbbell in front of you are particularly good for the gluteal muscles.

46. How can I train to prevent hip and thigh injuries?

Each femur fits into the pelvic (hip) girdle in a fairly deep socket. This is commonly called a ball-and-socket joint, but unlike the shoulder, extensive flexibility is not allowed due to the deep socket and fairly inflexible pelvic girdle. Anytime one is involved in standing, jumping, running, or landing, the hip and thigh are involved. When an injury occurs to this area, it seems like the whole body is affected since the hip and thigh are so central to the body. As discussed in Question 21, the common injuries to the hip and thigh are hamstring and groin strains, hip flexor strains, contusions to the thigh, and iliotibial band syndrome (ITBS).

Since the pelvic girdle is the origin of so many muscles above and below, stability of the pelvic girdle is very important. The exercises in Question 45 also stabilize the hips and are highly recommended. When standing on one leg, the hips resemble a suspension bridge. For example, if you are standing on your right foot, the left side of the pelvic girdle would collapse if a muscle on the outside of the right hip did not contract to prevent such a collapse. This is the purpose of the gluteus medius, a muscle that connects the outside of the pelvic girdle to the outside of the femur. Just standing is not a problem, but when running or landing on one foot, the gluteus medius must contract vigorously in order to keep the hips horizontal.

How to Strengthen the Gluteus Medius

A strong gluteus medius is critical for hip stability. Fortunately, this muscle is fairly easy to strengthen. A typical warm-up of the muscle is first recommended. Just lie on your side and raise your leg from the hip, keeping the leg straight. Roll over and lift the other leg. This is called hip abduction. To strengthen the gluteus medius, you can connect an elastic band to your leg and abduct your hip. Attach ankle weights to your leg and abduct your hip. Most fitness gyms have hip abduction machines. Another good strengthening exercise is to hop on one foot across a gym mat or grass. Increase the resistance by running and then hopping on one foot.

Hamstring Strain Prevention

As described in Question 21, hamstring tears are the bane of injuries for many sport participants. Hamstrings are often injured because they are biarticular muscles, affecting the hip and knee. When activity is intense, such as sprinting, accelerating, or turning quickly, synchronous hamstring activation is critical. Studies have shown that most hamstring injuries occur during the eccentric phase of sprinting. That is, the hamstring contracts but lengthens in order to slow down the rapidly extending knee. While this hamstring activity protects the knee joint, the hamstring is rapidly stretching and is vulnerable.

If the hamstring is injured while contracting eccentrically, one prevention strategy is to strengthen the hamstring eccentrically. The easiest way to do this is what some call the Russian hamstring exercise (also called the

Nordic hamstring exercise). Following a warm-up, kneel down on a mat or lawn with your body erect and arms crossed on your chest. Have a partner stabilize you at the ankle while you slowly lean forward from the knee, keeping your body in a straight line. As you move forward, you will feel stress in the hamstring, and at some point, the hamstring will begin to fail. Return to the upright position. Start off with one or two sets of 10 repetitions and increase the repetitions as you adapt. Keep in mind that this exercise will make you quite sore in the beginning. As you gain strength, you will be able to increase your range of motion before failure. As you get comfortable with this exercise, allow yourself to fall to the mat, catching yourself by the hands, and then push yourself back to the starting position.

Many people believe that extensive stretching of the hamstring prevents strains, but there is no sound evidence supporting this belief. Maintain moderate flexibility of the hamstrings using static and dynamic stretching on a regular basis. Warming up prior to vigorous activity is very important. Finally, since the activation of the hamstrings is so complicated during sprinting, fatigue is a factor. Fatigue affects control, so rest is needed between sprints to allow recovery.

Hip Flexor Injury Prevention

The hip flexors are located on the front of the hip and are highly recruited when running at higher speeds. Hip flexor strain is caused by overuse as well as acute injuries. Sprinting, kicking, and fast movements in racket sports are common causes. Hill running particularly stresses the hip flexors and is a good training method. Following a warm-up, sprint up a short hill, starting slowly and eventually moving to high speed. Keep in mind that this is not an endurance exercise, so the amount of time sprinting is only around 6–10 seconds. Running up a flight of stairs has a similar effect. Try running up every third step.

Groin Strain Prevention

Groin strains are slightly more common than hip flexor injuries and occur frequently to soccer and ice hockey players, breaststroke swimmers, and less frequently to football and basketball athletes. They are called groin strains because the injured muscles originate on the pubis. Breaststroke swimmers frequently experience groin pain, primarily caused by overuse. Studies have shown that breaststroke swimmers often try to swim through the pain. This doesn't work. Once the pain starts, there should be a reduction in breaststroke kicking until pain is gone; otherwise, the injury will worsen, requiring extensive rehabilitation and time to heal.

Groin strains to other athletes are mostly acute injuries, occurring when an abrupt, especially oblique, move is made. Since the groin muscles tend to adduct (pull the leg toward the middle) the leg, groin muscles need good strength. Researchers at Lennox Hill Hospital in New York found that a player was 17 times more likely to sustain a groin injury when the adductors were less than 80 percent the strength of the abductors. Flexibility was unrelated to injury. Subsequently, when at risk players were strengthened, the rate of injury went down. Clearly, strengthening the adductors is required. Many fitness gyms have hip adductor machines. An easy way to strengthen your adductors with little equipment is to use elastic bands. Attach the appropriate band to your ankle and adduct your leg while a partner is holding the band. You can do this in a sitting or standing position.

Preventing Iliotibial Band Syndrome

ITBS is an overuse injury causing pain to the outside of the knee. Like all overuse injuries, you cannot train through it. Continuing to train without change just results in a more serious strain. Maintaining the flexibility of the IT band is important, especially for people who tend to sit for much of the day and then go out and run. The typical IT band stretch: place your right foot behind you and to the left of your body while reaching over your head and to the right with your right hand. This is an exercise that can be easily done anywhere, so keeping the IT band flexible is not difficult.

Contusions to the Thigh

Contusions to the thigh are clearly acute injuries caused by tackling in football and rugby, high-speed impact with a ball or puck, or a misplaced kick in soccer. Athletes in football and ice hockey wear thigh pads to protect against contusions. Occasionally, athletes will leave these out, putting themselves at risk. Quadriceps contusions are hard to prevent, but immediate treatment is required to prevent further damage. The severity of quadriceps contusions is often underestimated since these often happen when the athlete is warm and motivated.

47. How do I stabilize my knee and reduce the frequency of knee injuries?

Question 22 presented the frequent injuries that occur to the knee joint. Other than wearing the appropriate shoes, shoes that do not adhere to the playing surface, there is little one can do to avoid injury due to contact. Most knee injuries, especially in sports other than football, are not the result of contact. These knee injuries occur during deceleration activities. Anytime an athlete lands, stops, or turns quickly, they decelerate. When the deceleration activity is uncontrolled, when the leg is too stiff or out of position, the leg can twist in an awkward position, causing injury. Research has shown that about 70 percent of anterior cruciate ligament (ACL) injuries occur in this manner—uncontrolled deceleration.

Although the knee is supported on both sides and in the interior by four ligaments, muscles provide significant stabilization to the knee. One key to knee stabilization is to have strong leg muscles that are also trained to stabilize the knee during deceleration. Drills designed to reduce impact forces and to maintain balance and control reduce knee injury. Considerable research has demonstrated that noncontact knee injuries can be reduced with proper training. Simple jumping drills reduce knee injury.

Strengthen Leg Muscles

Strength training for legs means multiple joint resistance exercises that are mostly done in a standing position. Various kinds of squats with barbells or dumbbells work well. Try one-legged squats, using hand supports when necessary. Training for leg stability often calls for putting one in an unstable position. One excellent way to do this is to squat on a Bosu balance trainer to strengthen and stabilize the lower legs. Try squatting on one leg on a Bosu while holding on to a support. Balance discs can also be used in a variety of ways while squatting.

Improve Landing Mechanics

Good landing mechanics means that the individual lands in a balanced position with their knees bent and directly over the feet. Many athletes tend to allow their knees to drift inwardly upon landing, thereby placing additional stress on medial knee ligaments. A good landing is also a quiet landing, a landing with a sequential flexing of ankle, knee, and hip. Such a landing reduces the impact forces, taking stress off knee ligaments. Although it is safer to land on two feet, athletes often land on one foot, placing themselves at additional risk. One foot landings should be practiced, focusing on balance and stability. In table 11, a set of landing drills one might use to improve landing mechanics is given. The goal of all these drills is a balanced quiet landing.

Table 11 Knee Stabilization Activities

Activity	Number/Time	Description
Wall jump	15 seconds	Perform repeated vertical jumps, landing in same spot without using arms
Tuck jumps	5–8	Repeated vertical jumps by swinging arms and bringing knees up to chest
Split jump	5–8	From the lunge position, jump straight up and switch legs. Repeat as quickly as possible.
One leg jumps	10	Jump off two feet as high as possible and land on one foot. Try not to move upon landing.
One leg jumps while travelling	5–8	From a mat or grass, jump forward off one foot, landing on the same foot. Repeat on other foot.
Lateral cone jumps	3 cones / 3 times	Hop sideways over three low cones with last jump on one foot—repeat
Lateral cone jumps—single leg*	3 cones / 3 times	Repeat but hop sideways on one leg—change legs and return
Quick side hops	15–20 seconds	Jump over and back a small cone or hurdle as quickly as possible
Quick side hops—one leg*	15–20 seconds	Repeat side hops on one leg—switch legs and repeat

*These jumps are more difficult and should not be done early in the program.

There are many variations one can add to these suggestions, but the basic recommendations remain—balanced and quiet landings are the goal. The preceding activities should be done two to three times per week, especially during a season.

Plyometric Exercises

Plyometric exercises are a great way to develop power (Question 41). In addition, plyometrics are very good at developing balance and knee stability. In the early stages of training, level plyometrics are recommended.

This means that each exercise starts and ends on the floor or mat. Progress to depth jumping, but make sure you are strong enough. If your legs tend to collapse upon landing, the box is too high.

Agility Training

Agility is the ability to change direction. Since turning is a deceleration activity, improving one's ability to change directions helps stabilize the knee. Agility training is fairly easy to set up; very little equipment is required, but one must be motivated to do agility training as fast as possible. Two things are important here: First, when the leg is straight, the tension on the ACL is greater. Therefore, try to bend at the knee when stopping and turning. Second, the hamstring muscles take the stress off the ACL. Therefore, agility exercises should involve a lot of backward movements, recruiting the hamstring muscles.

All you need to do agility training is to some way indicate where to change directions and a level surface. Most people use plastic cones, but anything works. Simply set up cones and a path that requires you to run forward, slide sideways left and right, stop and turn, and run backward. Allow enough rests between repetitions so that you can do this at full speed.

48. Are there specific ways to increase my ankle stability? What about ankle supports?

Sprained ankles are the most common injury in sport, accounting for 17 percent of soccer injuries and 25 percent of basketball injuries. Ankle sprains in volleyball are frequent, and almost always come from landing from a jump. Anytime one has to land or stop quickly, the ankle is at risk. Almost all ankle injuries are noncontact injuries resulting from an unbalanced landing or foot that is misplaced upon landing. Occasionally, an athlete comes down from a jump and lands on another player's foot. Most ankle sprains occur to the outside, the lateral side of the foot. Individuals with a history of ankle sprains are five times more likely to reinjure. Preventing the original ankle sprain is of prime importance. Fortunately, several practices have been developed to reduce the incidence of ankle sprains.

Footwear

People buy athletic footwear primarily based upon comfort as well as appearance. But improper footwear can result in a more susceptible athlete, especially if the shoes are too narrow. If the athlete's foot tends to bulge out the sides, the shoe is too narrow and less stable. Studies have shown that the soccer-style field shoe has the lowest incidence of ankle sprains. This shoe has fairly wide cleats (about 14) with a polyurethane sole. High-top shoes have the same injury frequency as low-cut shoes.

One aspect of footwear that affects injury is friction. Athletes need enough friction to start and stop, but too much friction amplifies the stopping force, placing the ankle, as well as the knee, at greater risk. Shoes do not have an independent friction score, but how the shoe moves across the surface does. For example, a soccer shoe will have a different tendency to slide horizontally on grass versus an artificial turf or dirt. Basketball and volleyball are typically played on wood floors, but not all wood floors are the same. In some gymnasiums, multiple groups play on floors all day. In such cases, any finish that was applied to the floor is worn off quickly. Friction is reduced as the year goes along. When possible, the shoe should be compatible with the surface.

Bracing

Ankle taping has been around as long as adhesive tape. Taping of ankles is just one form of providing external support to the ankle. Participants (usually not involved with a school team) have used a fairly simple fabric lace-up support. One of the benefits of these lace-up braces is that they can be tightened or loosened as necessary. It is well known that taping tends to loosen as a contest endures. Currently, there are a number of lace-up systems using various materials. One of these that has tested positively is the Swede-O universal lace-up ankle brace. Bilateral double-upright padded ankle braces are also fairly common in volleyball players.

Ankle taping remains very popular, but it is important that taping be done in a specific manner. When athletic trainers tape an ankle, they apply specific pressure to prevent inversion (turning inward) of the ankle. Unless you are quite skilled, this is difficult to do on yourself, and you are better off wearing a lace-up brace. It has been clearly shown that ankle taping works; the incidence of ankle sprains is lower for athletes playing with a taped ankle.

Balance and Proprioception Training

When a player lands from a jump on top of an opponent's foot, there is little you can do to prevent an ankle sprain. However, when landing with your foot misaligned, a landing that normally results in an ankle sprain, training helps. Proprioception refers to the body's ability to perceive its own position in space, like knowing the placement of the foot in the air. We perform many activities without having to stop and think. Proprioception relies on the relationship between the central nervous system and soft tissues such as muscles and tendons.

Proprioception can be improved. Proprioception can also be negatively affected by injury, one possible reason that injuries tend to repeat. A variety of activities can be introduced to help athletes with balance and proprioception. There are a lot of simple exercises one can use to improve proprioception and balance. The exercises described in Question 47 help with landing skills.

Research has found one effective training method to reduce ankle injuries in basketball. Balancing on a Wobble board, 16-inch round board with a 4-inch half sphere attached to the bottom, reduces ankle injury. The Wobble board is particularly good because it trains balance in 360° as opposed to balance boards that only balance in one plane. Start with simple balance drills like standing, then standing while passing or shooting a basketball, squatting, and then standing on one leg. Other skills can be used while balancing. Researchers had players practice five times a week in preseason and a shortened twice-a-week practice in season. Sessions were only about 10 minutes. Players who participated had a significant reduction in ankle injury.

Consider that an ankle injury can last for several weeks, possibly longer—that one ankle injury often leads to another. Participating in prevention techniques like 10 minutes of balance training does not take long, improves general conditioning of athletes, and reduces pain and suffering from injury.

49. How can I prevent a heat illness?

Question 25 describes the various heat illnesses. Since we create heat when we exercise, exercising in a hot environment, especially if the humidity is also high, presents a serious challenge. Consider the fact that the internal temperature of humans must stay within a fairly narrow range, increased body temperature, hyperthermia, can result in a range of illnesses including death. It is possible to exercise safely when the temperature rises, but this requires an increase in awareness and knowledge. Several strategies can be used to reduce the risk.

Assessment

How hot is it? That's the first question many people ask when they are concerned with the risk of a heat illness. Certainly the temperature of the ambient air is critical when determining risk, but insufficient when determining the full risk. The ambient air temperature does not help understand how easy it is to evaporate sweat, a primary heat loss system. Another aspect of assessment is the surface on which contests are played. Simply hearing the temperature on the radio station does not really tell us the temperature on the athletic field or the tennis court. It is well known that playing surfaces such as artificial turf or hard tennis surfaces result in increased ambient temperatures. Another factor is wind. Wind improves heat loss.

Use the heat index compiled by the National Weather Service to determine risk. The heat index takes into account the ambient temperature and the humidity. Humidity affects the rate of evaporation. Caution should be taken any time the heat index goes above 90 °F. One aspect of assessment missing in the heat index is radiation. When exercising in the sun, the body receives radiation that also increases heat, so if you are exercising on a sunny day, the risk may even be greater. Once an assessment has been made, you may want to modify your activity.

Modify Activity

When the risk of heat illness is high, modify your activity. Work out in early morning or around dusk. Remember that the activity you can do on a cool day may be too intense on a hot day. Unless you are highly acclimated, your ability to exercise is compromised in the heat, so reduce the intensity; save it for a cooler day. Long continuous work is going to be more difficult, so break up the workout frequently, taking time to rest and hydrate.

Acclimatization

Fortunately, regular exercise in a warm environment results in physiological adaptations. Blood flow improves, sweating improves, and there is less loss of electrolytes in the sweat. Acclimatization takes about 10 days, but some people take longer. During the acclimatization period, exercise should be vigorous but not overwhelming. A gradual increase in work results in the best acclimatization. Occasionally, people will travel to a hot environment to participate in an event. In such cases, individuals usually do not have time to acclimatize to the location, so acclimatization to the heat must be done before the trip. If your environment is not normally hot, you will need to create an artificial hot space. Wearing extra clothing is one strategy, but you can turn up the heat in a room and cycle or run on a treadmill.

Wear Appropriate Clothing

There are two reasons that so many heat illnesses occur in football: the football uniform and helmet reduce the ability to evaporate sweat, and football often starts in late summer. The football uniform compromises sweat evaporation. Fortunately, many high school and college federations have mandated an acclimatization period during which athletes train without the football uniform. One important clothing factor in hot environments is the ability of sweat to evaporate. There appears to be no the best material that research has identified, but materials should be thin and fit well. In many situations, the best practice is to have the skin exposed. If it is sunny out, a light-colored hat is a good option, but evaporation from the head should be facilitated, so take off your helmet or hat when resting in the shade. In general, lighter colored clothing does not absorb radiation.

Hydration

For years, coaches and athletes believed that drinking water during exercise sessions was not a good idea, that water consumption would make you sick. Today, water consumption during exercise is the norm as exercise scientists have found that adequate hydration provides a strong defense of heat stress. Also, hydrated athletes perform better. During exercise, some dehydration is to be expected. For example, very large football athletes can lose 10–15 pounds of fluid during a long intense practice. A gallon of water weighs 8 pounds, requiring some athletes to drink as much as 2 gallons! Hydration involves a three-fold approach:

- Prehydration: One goal is to start practice or competition with normal water content. About four hours before practice or competition, the athlete should slowly drink the amount of fluid listed in table 12 according to body weight.
- During Practice: Water or supplemental beverages should be readily available, cool, and palatable. Try frequent small breaks rather than one big break.

Table 12 Pre-Activity Fluid Intake Suggestions

Body Weight (lbs.)	Fluid (ounces)
110	8.5–12
132	10–14
154	12–16.5
176	13.5–19
198	15–21
220	17–24
242	18.5–26
264	20–28.5
286	22–31

- Postexercise: Since it is almost impossible to replace all the fluid when exercising, athletes need to pay attention to replacing fluids and electrolytes postexercise. Besides drinking fluids, eating foods and snacks that are high in water and sodium is helpful. Replacement beverages should include carbohydrates and electrolytes, but the carbohydrate concentration should be fairly low.

Considerable research (often supported by Gatorade) has been conducted on exercise beverages. Keep in mind that you do not have to replace all lost fluids and fuels with a postexercise beverage. People normally eat between exercise sessions, adding fuels, electrolytes, and water. One recommendation that is easy to follow is to just drink water when the exercise session is less than an hour, but choose some sort of replacement beverage for longer sessions.

Hyponatremia

Some years back, a radio talk show host encouraged a group of women to enter a competition to win a prize for one of their children. The woman who drank the most ended up in the hospital and died of hyponatremia. Staying hydrated is healthy, but drinking more than one needs is unnecessary and occasionally dangerous. Hyponatremia is a disorder in fluid-electrolyte balance that results in an abnormally low plasma sodium concentration, causing a disruption in the osmotic balance in the blood–brain barrier. This causes an influx of water into the brain, possibly causing a fatal response. In one study of 330 triathletes, about 18 percent showed signs of hyponatremia. About one-third required hospitalization. Excessive water consumption should be avoided.

50. How can I avoid common injuries while running, cycling, and skiing?

Sport injuries can happen in any sport, but three popular fitness and recreational activities require specific interest. Millions of people jog, bike, and ski every year but with mixed results. Most participate without injury and enjoy the benefits of regular exercise. Indeed, these are all great activities, but injury can ruin one's favorite pastime. As discussed earlier, some injuries result in cessation of activity, a significant loss. An educated approach to these activities reduces injury.

Jogging

Jogging remains one of the most popular aerobic activities. The incidence of individuals getting hurt while jogging is still debated, but there is no question that many are hurt while jogging. Throughout this text, there has been a consistent position that the body adapts to stress through a process of fatigue and recovery. Too much stress, too little recovery, or a combination of the two often leads to injury.

Jogging is not for everyone; some people are better off choosing an aerobic program other than running. People who are very overweight, have chronic knee problems, or foot problems will encounter have fewer injuries if they participate in an activity in which the body is supported. Cycling, rowing, and swimming are all supported activities, placing less stress on knees and ankles. Walking might be the better option. With the advent of various elliptical machines often found in fitness gyms, you can participate in an aerobics program that is not as stressful on knees, ankles, and hips.

Start slowly.

- Let's say you've decided to start jogging. Unfortunately, if you have a desk job, sit most of the day, you're not ready. First, try some vigorous walking four to five times a week for a mile or two for the first couple of weeks. Next, start interspersing short jogging intervals into the walking program. For example, run 10 steps and then walk 10 steps. You don't need to exhaust yourself; you are slowly getting your body to adapt. Once this feels comfortable, try 20 steps, then 30, and so on.

Continue to use interval training of this nature for about 6 weeks. Be patient but consistent.

- Intersperse rest days with work days. During the early days of running, run only three to four days a week.
- Increase mileage slowly. The 10% rule is your guide to increasing mileage. Once you have become comfortable, you may want to increase your mileage. The rule is to increase no more than 10 percent a week.
- Once you have achieved a regular running program, be satisfied. You cannot increase indefinitely, so find that reasonable workout and maintain.
- Footwear is important and should only be worn for jogging. It's better to get professional support from a running shop to purchase running shoes. Do you have excess pronation or supination? Just look at the bottom of a worn pair of shoes and see how it is worn. Show this to the salesperson.
- Maintain good hip and core strength. The muscles for running originate on your pelvic girdle, so this part of the body must be stable enough to support running. McGill's Big 3 listed in the "Directory of Resources" will help with this.
- Listen to your body. Trust your intuition when creating and maintaining a running program (or any program). Each person is so individualized that no one source can tell you exactly what to do. If something feels wrong, then it is. You cannot run through pain; it won't get better.

Cycling

Bicycling is a great sport, but it is also one of the more dangerous sports. About 1,000 people die a year from bicycle accidents, and there are about half-million bicycle injuries a year. Every bicycle manual insists that cyclists must wear a helmet, and some states have even mandated helmets. Helmets should fit and should be certified. The fact remains that helmets do not prevent collisions with cars, the principal cause of bicycle deaths. "Obey the law" is another common suggestion, but obeying the law is not enough as you can easily get run over by a car even though you are obeying the law. How can we prevent collisions with cars?

- Ride on the right side of the road.
- Ride in the bike lane when you can. This is a no-brainer, but if there is no bike lane, you would want cars to go around you. This means you ride in the car lane but on the right.

- Do not ride too far to the right. Yes, you are obeying the law but also vulnerable to someone opening their car door. If you're too far to the right, you cannot often be seen by parked motorists or by people pulling out from a car parking lot or a side street.
- Ride to be visible. Riding just off the right fender of a car is a blind spot. A driver can take a quick right turn and never see you. When approaching an intersection, look directly at the driver in the incoming traffic. Wave or raise your hand if they don't see you.
- Do not ride on the sidewalk.
- Light up. Lights are cheap, but many cyclists don't wear them even at night. Wear clothing that has reflective strips.
- Forget music players and phones. If you need to use your phone, pull over and stop.
- Avoid busy streets.
- Signal when you turn.
- Use a mirror.

Interest in mountain biking has increased tremendously. Bike parks have opened all over the country that support trail riding. Mountain bikes are different, allowing riders to ride in a more upright position. Mountain bikes often have suspension systems, and good brakes are critical. Mountain bikers don't have to worry about cars, but they do have to watch other riders as well as the terrain. Spills are not that unusual, so riders need to learn to safely fall. Some riders use clips, but this is probably not a good idea for novice riders. Riders need to learn how to get off and on quickly.

Riding in large groups is not a good idea on mountain biking trails. Obey the rules of the facility. In many areas, there are clear trails that are only for uphill or downhill riders. Riding the wrong way is analogous to riding the wrong way on a one-way street. Don't overrate your ability. Just because you ride a bike on the road doesn't mean you are ready for trails.

Downhill Skiing

Just a short time back, a helmeted recreational skier was fairly uncommon. Today, many skiers wear helmets designed for downhill skiing. Helmets are highly recommended for riders who ski off trail or participate in glade skiing. While glade skiing is particularly attractive, it is not for novices. Glade skiing requires skiers to make quick controlled turns. Snow conditions vary more in glades, so skiers need to adjust quickly.

Other than a good ski helmet, the bindings and skis are especially important. The ski should fit your skill level, so be honest when you are describing your ability when purchasing equipment. Your face is particularly vulnerable to frostbite, so plan to cover it if necessary. If you start to get frostbite while skiing, it's not going to go away if you keep skiing. Once you have developed frostbite spots, it's best to get off the mountain and try another day. Watch for ice, especially in certain areas of the country that tend to have less snow.

The FIS (International Ski Federation) has established rules that all skiers should follow:

- Respect other skiers and snowboarders. Act so that you do not endanger others.
- Control your speed.
- Choose your route so that you do not endanger people in front of you.
- When overtaking another skier, give them enough room to make their turns; don't get too close.
- When entering a marked trail or starting after taking a quick stop, look up and down the mountain before starting.
- Unless absolutely necessary, a skier should avoid stopping on the piste (the trail) when the trail is narrow or visibility is restricted. When falling in such a place, clear the area as soon as possible.
- If climbing or descending on foot, stay to the side of the piste.
- Respect all signs and markings.
- Skiers are duty bound to assist others when there is an accident.
- Skiers must exchange names and addresses following an accident.

Skiing injuries are also prevented by preparation. Skiing is tough on the lower body, so get in shape before you go out. The suggestions in Questions 45 and 46 for strengthening back, hip, and knee should be followed. The first few trips of the year are more vulnerable. You can't start off where you ended the year before, and you're going to fatigue quicker. Fatigue is a common cause of injury, so take more breaks than usual, allowing you to get in shape.

Case Studies

1. MELISSA HAS MULTIPLE ACL SURGERIES

Melissa was one of the most promising soccer athletes in northern Michigan. Her soccer skills were a pleasure to watch, and she was tough. Playing regularly with her three older brothers, she knew how to fight for the ball. Melissa was good, the best player in her high school. In her junior year, her school won the state championship, and Melissa was voted most valuable player. College coaches were contacting her; her goal was a Division 1 (D1) soccer scholarship.

Melissa was looking forward to her senior year, but she had a new coach. The new coach was different; she had read somewhere that soccer players can run up to seven miles in a game. The new coach used this finding to set up a running program for the soccer players. That summer, Melissa started the coach's running program, running 20–25 miles a week. Fall practice started, and the distance running continued, but Melissa felt like she had lost some of her speed; her legs were tired. In the third game of the season, she went up for a header, bumped into her opponent, and landed awkwardly on her left leg. She heard a "pop" and went down. She knew she was hurt, but she was able to get up and walk off the field. That night while eating dinner, she turned slightly, and she felt like her knee actually dislocated. It seemed to lock, but she moved it around a bit, and the feeling resolved. She knew something was seriously wrong.

Lying in the MRI tube for what seemed forever, she worried. She met the next day with the orthopedic surgeon and learned the bad news: torn anterior cruciate ligament (ACL), torn MCL, torn medial meniscus—the Unhappy Triad. She was told to go home, ice regularly, sign up for physical therapy, and get ready for surgery. She went to physical therapy, and her leg got better. She could walk without limping; her leg didn't collapse, but she knew it wasn't right.

In the hospital two weeks later, the doctor explained the surgery; he would take a piece of her patella tendon to replace the ACL and also take out the small piece of torn meniscus. "Don't worry, you will be good as new," he said. The night after surgery was tough: no sleep, pain, worries. Melissa went home the next day on crutches. Physical therapy started. Her therapist told her she had had the same surgery, but she was very encouraging. "There are going to be some ups and downs, but you will be back." Melissa was very motivated and ready to work, and she did. After nine months, she felt she was ready to play again.

Melissa had an excellent soccer history but a strike against her. Coaches knew she was vulnerable, but most coaches were familiar with ACL injuries, and only a few didn't have at least one player who didn't have an ACL tear. Finally, Melissa got a D1 scholarship offer. It wasn't a top program or one she wanted, but she wanted to play college soccer. Arriving on campus in late summer, she quickly became friends with most of the players, and she was happy to be on a team again. The season started, but it had been a year since any competition and she started slowly. But soon she adapted; she was vigorous, aggressive, and skilled. She was back.

Sophomore year started, and it was the fourth game when a player charged right at her, faked, and Melissa twisted her leg one way and her body went the other. Another ACL tear of the same leg, another surgery, and another rehabilitation. Melissa fought back, but it was harder the second time. Her injured leg didn't look the same. She returned for her junior year, but she was no longer the star. It wasn't lack of effort; her leg just didn't feel the same. She thought back to the words of the surgeon and knew he was wrong. "I'm not as good as new."

Following graduation, she and four of her friends decided to take the trip they had always discussed, biking across country. They started off in Boston on June 1, heading west. During a rest day in Utah, they camped near a high school. A soccer game was going on, and Melissa decided to step in. Melissa knew she wasn't in soccer shape, but this was low-level competition, and she felt she could do it. She couldn't. ACL tear #3.

The third surgery failed, and the doctor wasn't sure whether a fourth would work. Today, Melissa is living in Florida, teaching and coaching high school soccer. She cannot run and walks with a limp. She is 29. Her orthopedic surgeon says she is a good candidate for a knee replacement.

Analysis

Soccer players do run up to seven miles in a game, but none of the running is continuous. Continuous running does not prepare you for soccer. During a game, soccer players walk, jog, sprint briefly, stop, turn, and jump. During her early years, Melissa's coaches trained her just for that. Playing with her brothers in the backyard also facilitated these same skills. Although Melissa didn't specifically do any knee stabilization exercises, the constant play helped.

Melissa's ability to play soccer was compromised by the continuous running. Not only had she slowed, but she had also lost some of her coordination and speed. The slow running had diminished Melissa's fast-twitch fibers, the fibers needed for quick stabilization. In the United States, there are multiple soccer organizations providing excellent instruction about appropriate training and injury prevention. But coaches have to attend. Further, coaches have to prepare to change—that anecdotal information is not research. Melissa's college coach had seen FIFA's manual oriented to warm-up and injury prevention, but he felt that it would take too much time away from soccer. Would Melissa have gotten hurt the second time if she had participated in such a program? No one can answer this, but the evidence is clear that these programs work. They reduce the incidence of injury.

Melissa made a big mistake playing in the pickup soccer game. After spending weeks on the bicycle, there was no way she was prepared for soccer. Coupled with a history of two ACL reconstructions was her downfall. Recovering from three reconstructions is difficult at best. The failure rate of reconstructions increases with multiple reconstructions.

2. YOLANDA GETS STRESS FRACTURES

Yolanda grew up in the shadow of her big sister, Jesse. Four years older, Jesse was the best runner in her school, and Yolanda wanted to be just like her. Occasionally, Jesse would invite Yolanda along for a run. Yolanda could keep up, but just barely. Yolanda's stride was a little awkward at first, but she started to get smoother and smoother. Jesse encouraged her to go out for the cross-country team when she got to junior high. Seventh grade started and Yolanda joined the cross-country team. She loved the freedom of running trails and quickly moved to the top of the ladder. It was Jesse who cheered her on when Yolanda broke her junior high record.

The local college-sponsored winter track meets every Friday, and Yolanda starting competing in the mile run. Schools from all over competed; it was loud and it was fun. She learned to be a strategic runner, saving herself for that final kick. People started noticing her, even though she was only 12. That spring, she ran outdoor track and continued to improve.

Eighth grade started, and the coach moved Yolanda up to the varsity. She was now competing along with her sister. She couldn't beat Jesse, but they were a formidable pair; the school paper called them "the dynamite duo." They both ran winter track and continued that spring. It was the last meet of the year; Jesse was graduating when they came in first and second in the mile. Yolanda ran a mile in 5:10, the state record for girls under 14.

Yolanda took the summer off from running as the family took a cross-country vacation to celebrate Jesse's graduation and track scholarship to the state university. Yolanda started cross-country, but she wasn't in her best shape. The coach told her that if she lost a few pounds she could run the hills better. Yolanda started cutting back on meals and would jump rope every night in the basement. She felt the pressure of living up to her sister's reputation. She lost weight, but it wasn't long before she stopped menstruating. She didn't say anything to anyone about it. Her running was going well.

During winter track, she started feeling a sharp pain in her foot. At first, the pain went away when she stopped running, but before long it hurt most of the time. The school athletic trainer thought she had a stress fracture, and the doctor confirmed a stress fracture in her third metatarsal. She put Yolanda in a walking boot to take the stress off her foot. Yolanda did not do anymore jump rope, but she watched her weight, often pretending to eat more. She took her lunch to school but never ate it, sharing it with her friends. She got a gym membership and cycled endlessly on an indoor cycle.

Yolanda spent six difficult weeks in the walking boot. She was happy to have maintained her weight. She had not regained her menstrual cycle. Even with all the cycling, when she looked at herself in the mirror she could see the atrophy in her injured leg. But she was ready to start running again. Track season was coming up. She started training again and followed the trainer's suggestion to take it slow. But this only lasted for a while, and she was back to full speed, adding some jump rope to her running program. About halfway through the spring season, she started feeling pain again, this time in her shin—the diagnosis: stress fracture of the tibia. This time the physician put a cast on her lower leg and assigned her crutches.

Yolanda was crushed, depressed. Eventually, she confessed to her mother that she had not had a period in a year. Her mother took her to a gynecologist who was concerned about Yolanda's weight and amenorrhea. Yolanda told the doctor that the loss of running would make her fat. Her doctor suggested that Yolanda get some counseling to deal with her depression and weight concerns. Yolanda responded well to the counselor, confessing that she had been hiding her meals. Her mother also had her meet with a nutritionist who gave Yolanda some good advice. Within a few months, Yolanda had regained her menstrual cycle and felt good about her body. She took the summer off from running and is ready for the cross-country season.

Analysis

For many years, the common belief was that the loss of one's menstrual period, amenorrhea, was not that serious. The research was primarily based upon whether the ability to conceive later would be affected. The loss of one's period during the teenage years did not seem to affect the ability to get pregnant later. The problem is more related to the development of bone density as opposed to child bearing. Bone is in a constant state of growth and replacement. During growth is when Yolanda would be developing her bone density. Once mature, an increase in bone density is minimal if at all. It is critically important that Yolanda reach her maximum bone density. The loss of a regular cycle compromises her bone density, making her much more susceptible to osteoporosis later in life.

Yolanda's loss of her regular menstrual cycle could be related to a host of factors. Certainly, the loss of weight and possible malnutrition is a factor. The extra exercise, especially rope skipping, is another factor. Poor nutrition and excess exercise is an energy drain on any individual and robs one of their normal development. All of this coupled with the stress of competition and living up to her sister's record were factors. Finally, the coach's suggestion that she might be a little overweight was a big mistake.

Fortunately, Yolanda admitted to her mother about her amenorrhea, and her mother handled it properly. The therapist and the nutritionist helped get her back to a normal healthy cycle. Unfortunately, this is a problem that affects many young women. Many have the belief that a lost cycle is not a problem, that it will return at some point. As well, some are relieved that they don't have to deal with it. Long-term bone health is critically important, and a normal eumenorrheic cycle is one key to healthy bone.

3. JERRY BURNS OUT ON TENNIS

When Jerry was little, his dad put up a tennis backboard in the driveway, gave him a racket and a few balls, and let him play. Jerry loved hitting the ball, especially after he stopped hitting it over the backboard. He just loved pounding away at the ball. He and a couple of his friends developed their own game, a type of handball using tennis rackets. Other boys started coming around, and Jerry got better and better. He was clearly the best player, even with boys who were older.

Jerry's dad started taking an interest in the game. He could see how good Jerry was and wanted to support him. The local recreational program sponsored tennis clinics, and Jerry's dad signed him up. Playing on a full court was fun. Jerry's driveway skills transferred to the big court, and he learned quickly. The coach taught him how to serve; he was a natural. Jerry turned 10 that summer and played in the end of summer tournament. Jerry won his age group, 10 and under, tournament.

Jerry continued playing some tennis throughout the year at the local college. They had an indoor tennis facility and offered classes to local youth on weekends. His game flourished, and his dad felt that Jerry could go far in tennis. That summer, he sent Jerry off to a tennis camp for a month. Upon arriving, Jerry realized that some of the boys had actually been coming to this camp since they were eight. Most were better than Jerry but not for long as the competition was just what he needed.

Upon returning home, Jerry's dad signed him up with a private tennis coach. Jerry played tennis every day throughout the year. He started traveling to tournaments, started winning more, and soon became one of the better players in the Gulf States. Jerry's dad attended every match, often videotaping the games and analyzing them afterward. At 13, he lost in the finals at the Gulf States tournament. He was determined to win next year.

Jerry continued working; tennis was his only sport. The next summer he made it to the 14 and under finals of the Gulf States tennis championship. He was the number 1 seed and expected to win. He had already beaten his opponent before. But he was tired; his body was sore and his elbow was tender. He was having trouble sleeping. His usual drive was just not there. He lost in straight sets. His dad was furious. He had invested so much.

After the tournament ended, he went out to practice, but his elbow and wrist were hurting. His physical therapist taught him a set of exercises for his elbow, but his main advice was that Jerry needed some time off from tennis. The therapist convinced his dad he needed rest.

During his time off, he picked up a book detailing the lives of several prominent athletes. He read that Peyton and Eli Manning only played football in the backyard of their home until high school. Joe Namath played football, basketball, and baseball in a seasonal manner. Namath was offered a baseball contract but decided to play football. Bruce Jenner didn't even specialize in track until he was finishing high school. None of these great athletes only played one sport until they were older. Jerry loved tennis, but he also wanted to play a team sport, joining in with his peers.

He joined the junior varsity basketball team and loved the camaraderie of a team. Playing with the other boys reminded him of his old games in the driveway. He was having fun. His coach also started the boys on a strength training program. Jerry had never done any of this. His tennis coach thought weight training would hurt his tennis. When basketball season ended, Jerry continued to strength train. Later that spring, he decided to hit a few balls on the tennis court. His wrist and elbow pain were gone. He was rested, bigger and stronger. It felt good to hit the ball again. "Maybe I'll play in the Gulf States next year," he said to himself. "I need to play some basketball this summer."

Analysis

Jerry's story is typical of how outside pressures can turn a playful activity into something resembling a job. This is especially true if the pressure is coming from a parent. Typically, children want to please their parents and will go along. Meanwhile, parents often have the mistaken belief that if a child doesn't start sport early, they will not reach top-level form. Parents also see achievement in sport as the pathway to a college scholarship and sport fame.

Jerry loved tennis, but it became more of a chore than fun. Playing an individual sport is often socially isolating. Combining schoolwork with the rigors of daily tennis practice removed Jerry from many of the normal social activities. Fortunately, Jerry received good advice from his physical therapist, and his dad accepted this. In many cases, this is not the usual response as parents have invested so much in their children—too much pride and pleasure from their achievement. Children can also become involved in this trap, that winning is the only way to their parent's love.

Studies conducted by the Canadian Sport for Life group have shown that specialization at an early age is not necessary for high-level achievement. Sampling multiple sports and activities is highly recommended for youth, and that specialization should not start early. Further, children who specialize tend to burn out, often quitting the sport altogether. Certainly, the system fails when what starts out as a fun backyard game ends up becoming tiresome.

Fortunately, Jerry has not lost his love for sport. He has learned new skills and got new friends, and he will probably return to the tennis court with renewed promise. Weight training has not hurt his tennis.

4. LUKE DECIDES TO GET A SECOND OPINION

Luke started weight training when he was 13. His dad was a physical education teacher at the high school and taught Luke how to safely lift. Luke loved the challenge of weight training and kept at it. He received support at home, but elsewhere people questioned his activity. "Doesn't weight lifting at your age stunt your growth?" Luke's dad assured him that a careful program was good for him and that weight training was a good idea. It worked. Luke got stronger and stronger, bench pressing over 300 pounds when he was only 16.

Luke finished high school. At 6 feet and 180 pounds, weight training had not stunted his growth; he was the tallest person in his family. Luke went to college and earned a degree in kinesiology and a master's in nutrition. He took a job at the local community college teaching health and wellness courses and directing the fitness gym.

Luke loved the gym; working with students interested in health and fitness was very rewarding. He continued with his strength training program, but he dropped heavy weight lifting. He developed his own resistance program using a combination of body weight exercises, dumbbell and kettle ball training, and mobility exercises. He didn't do excessive strengthening of only one body part. He understood the need for symmetry.

Mountain biking was his second passion. One day he was going on a steep downhill when his front tire caught a tree root and threw him to the ground. He hit his shoulder hard, but Luke didn't think it was too bad. He couldn't sleep on that shoulder during the night, and the next day at the gym he found that anything he did overhead was painful. He decided he needed to see an orthopedic surgeon. His dad told him to get ready for surgery. "After all, isn't that what they do?"

The surgeon diagnosed his problem as a torn labrum, and the subsequent MRI confirmed it. The orthopedist recommended surgery. Luke was concerned. He had just watched his dad recover from surgery on his rotator cuff—five weeks in a sling tied to his body. A friend of Luke's had labrum surgery and had still not recovered. Luke decided to see another surgeon. She said surgery might be necessary, but let's first try a conservative approach, physical therapy.

Luke went to the local hospital for therapy. He was assigned a therapist who put him through the usual tests and started with therapy. Luke was slowly improving but wasn't too optimistic. One day his original therapist wasn't there, and he met with another therapist. The approach was very different, and the therapist put him through some exercises that Luke had never done. During the session, Luke realized that the new therapist specialized in shoulder injuries. His dad suggested he switch therapists, and Luke made the request. He felt better already. Twice a week, Luke met with the therapist, and he was tenacious at home, performing all the exercises regularly. Luke reviewed his old textbooks on shoulder anatomy and analyzed each exercise.

After eight weeks of training, Luke had regained all of his range of motion and most of his strength. He still had a little trouble with some movements. High-speed overhand throwing bothered him some, but not enough to risk surgery. A follow-up meeting with his orthopedic surgeon was positive. Her only recommendation was that Luke continue the shoulder mobility and strengthening exercises. "Just maintain your current conditioning and you will be fine. Once a week is all you need."

Analysis

Luke was fortunate that he had a dad to help with advice. All too often when people encounter some sport injury, they think first of surgery. The media is full of stories of athletes begin carted off the field directly to the operating room. In many cases, this might be the necessary form of treatment, but not always. What might be the routine treatment for the professional athlete may not be what is recommended for everyone. Professional athletes get paid for performance, and they want to get back as soon as possible. A longer duration conservative approach does not often suit them.

Luke had seen how tough it was for his dad to recover from shoulder surgery. Further, his friend had already had labrum surgery and had not recovered. It wasn't that Luke was particularly afraid of surgery; he wasn't ready to jump right into it. Getting the second opinion was the best thing he did under the circumstance. If the second surgeon had said the surgery was necessary, he would have done it. But there was no real rush. Luke wasn't in a great deal of pain and had the time to devote to therapy.

Many people refrain from getting a second opinion. Some are worried that the original doctor will not approve. Some don't want to take the time, but Luke had the time and did the right thing. Luke also learned that not all physical therapists are the same. The shoulder is a very complicated joint, and not every therapist knows it well. Luke was assigned to the first available therapist. Fortunately, he found one more knowledgeable, and his dad suggested he switch.

Luke has had a very successful treatment. His orthopedist has recommended that Luke continue to maintain good shoulder mobility and strength. This advice is very common but often not followed. People often stop doing the thing that actually made them well. Everyone knows that in order to keep a car running well, you have to maintain it. The same is true for the body; maintaining your fitness is relatively easy. You just have to do it.

5. BRYAN SUFFERS SECOND IMPACT SYNDROME

Bryan had it all. He came from a wealthy family, lived in a great neighborhood, and had his own car. At 6 feet 1 inch and 210 pounds, he was a force to be feared on the football field. Bryan was also a very good student, and he worked hard and was confident of his future. Football practice started in August, and the two-a-day practices were tough. But Bryan believed that the camaraderie and the Friday Night Lights were worth it. Bryan's coach believed he needed to instill toughness in his players; head-on tackling was his answer. Players were placed 10 yards apart; one was the ball carrier and one was the tackler. They ran straight into each other. The players hated it; they also knew that this kind of tackling rarely happened in a game. Bryan didn't like the drill, but he didn't avoid it either; linebackers need to tackle.

Bryan lined up; he was the tackler. Wham! Bryan's head snapped back as the runner's elbow hit him on the jaw. Bryan made the tackle; he was able to get up but had trouble maintaining his balance. He was very dizzy. "You got your bell rung," said the smiling coach. Fortunately, the drill was over, and the practice soon ended. Bryan went into the locker room and threw up. His head was killing him. He made it home but felt terrible; his head hurt, and he was a little dizzy and nauseous. Over the weekend, he recovered a little. School started the following Monday. Thankfully, two-a-day practices were over.

Bryan went to practice on Monday afternoon. He was afraid to tell the coach or the athletic trainer, as their first game was Friday night. Practice started off reasonably well, but Monday practices were always full contact. Bryan knew he wasn't himself. About halfway through practice, Bryan went to tackle the big fullback, and their helmets met. Bryan got up, walked around a bit, and fell over. Two days later, he woke up in the intensive care unit of the hospital. He tried to speak but couldn't, and there seemed to be tubes everywhere. He didn't know where he was and didn't remember anything.

Bryan stayed in intensive care for four more days and was moved to a rehabilitation unit. It took another week before Bryan could walk, even with support. The noises around him all seemed way too loud. His speech was still a bit slurred, but he was coming around. Six weeks later, he left the hospital. He still didn't remember any of the events leading up to his second concussion. Returning to school was tough. The sounds were so loud, and he was having trouble concentrating. Schoolwork seemed so difficult.

Bryan couldn't stay in school; he was depressed and cried occasionally without any real reason. He was so uncomfortable around the other kids; everything seemed to be happening at high speed. He often became dizzy just walking to class. He couldn't sit still long enough to do work, much less pass a test. He had lost 20 pounds, and his clothes didn't fit. His old confidence was gone. He continued with rehabilitation, slowly improving. At home, he spent a lot of time on the couch, dozing and watching television. Reading was difficult. Six months after the accident, he was able to jog for five minutes on the treadmill. Everyone gathered round to support him.

Bryan returned to school in the fall. Many of his buddies had graduated, but he was welcomed. He was still a shell of his former self. He weighed 180 pounds and wasn't very muscular. He walked slower than most and spoke a bit slower. He was getting by in school, but he had to work much harder. He graduated from high school that May and entered the local community college in the fall. He has no desire to play football, but he's getting better.

Analysis

Bryan suffered "second impact syndrome" (SIS), which is a term used to describe how the brain swells rapidly when a person suffers a second concussion before symptoms from an earlier concussion have subsided. Most concussion symptoms last about 7–10 days, but some are longer. The fact that Bryan had his second concussion within three days was very problematic. Actually Bryan was one of the lucky ones, as some studies show that SIS is fatal for about 90 percent of recipients. Unfortunately, many SIS patients have symptoms that don't go away. Chronic fatigue, headaches, and ambulatory problems can last forever.

The head-on tackling drill that the coach liked is a poor choice. Not only does it place athletes at excessive risk, but the drill also does not replicate what actually happens on the football field. When Bryan got up from his first concussion, he was dizzy. That symptom should have set off a chain of events orchestrated by the coach and the athletic trainer to identify if Bryan had suffered a concussion. Bryan was smart; he should have known that the additional symptoms he had from his first concussion were serious. But athletes do not normally pursue this information independently. It is the responsibility of the coach and the sports medicine staff to thoroughly educate students about concussion symptoms. Athletes must trust that reporting symptoms does not result in punitive action.

The future that Bryan foresaw will not happen. SIS is catastrophic, and Bryan will probably have some ill effects throughout his life. Certainly, the athletic future he anticipated is gone. His cognitive ability has been impaired.

Unfortunately, in the United States most states and programs do not require coaches to have an academic background specific to practicing healthy athletics. Too often, coaches receive their positions simply by being athletes, often perpetuating unsafe practices. Many head coaches insist that their assistants learn enough sports medicine to practice safely, but many do not. All too often, the emphasis is exclusively on how to win games. The coach has the ultimate responsibility for the health and safety of their athletes. Being unaware of how to practice healthy athletics is a dereliction of duty.

Glossary

ACL: anterior cruciate ligament. The ACL is the small ligament connecting the anterior part of the tibia to the posterior femur.

Amenorrhea: the absence of menstruation or one or more missed menstrual periods. Women who have missed at least three menstrual periods in a row are considered to have amenorrhea.

Anterior Cruciate Ligament: see ACL.

Arthroscope: the device used in arthroscopic surgery. Arthroscopy is a minimally invasive surgical procedure in which a treatment of damage is performed using an arthroscope.

Articular cartilage: the cartilage at the end of all bones that articulate with another bone. Articular cartilage protects bone and when damaged can result in osteoarthritis.

Atrophy: the reduction in size of a muscle due to disuse. Atrophy begins soon after a limb is immobilized in a cast or brace.

Avulsion Fracture: an injury to the bone in a location where a tendon or ligament attaches to the bone. When an avulsion fracture occurs, the tendon or ligament pulls off a piece of the bone.

Body Dysmorphia: is a mental disorder in which an individual is preoccupied by a small disorder that others cannot even see.

Bursitis: a painful condition that affects the fluid filled sacs, bursae, which protect soft tissues especially around joints.

Concussion: a traumatic brain injury that affects brain function. Repeated concussions may lead to long-term brain problems.

CTE: Chronic traumatic encephalopathy (CTE) is a progressive degenerative disease of the brain found in people with a history of repetitive brain traumas.

Epiphysis: the rounded end of a bone below which growth occurs—the epiphyseal plate.

Eumenorrhea: a healthy normal menstrual cycle usually recurring every 21–45 days.

Exercise Addiction: an unhealthy obsession with physical fitness and exercise. It is occasionally associated with distorted body image and eating disorders.

Fasciotomy: a surgical procedure where the fascia is cut to relieve tension or pressure in an area of the body to prevent loss of circulation. Fasciotomy is often used to treat acute compartment syndrome.

Female Triad: an interrelationship disorder including menstrual dysfunction, low energy (often caused by an eating disorder), and reduced bone density.

Fibula: the smaller bone on the outside of the shin.

Groin Strain: a strain of those muscles that originate near the pubis. These muscles are responsible for adduction (bringing the leg inward) of the femur.

High Ankle Sprain: a sprain that involves a different set of ligaments than the common ankle sprain. These ligaments are located above the ankle joint and between the tibia and fibula. A high ankle sprain takes longer to heal.

Hypertrophy: the increase in muscle mass often connected to strength training.

Hyponatremia: a serious condition that occurs when your sodium level is too low, causing cells to swell. It can occur by drinking too much water.

Iliotibial Band Syndrome: also called ITBS or ITband. An overuse injury to the connective tissue on the lateral side of the leg.

Impingement: occurs when there is **impingement** of tendons or bursa in the shoulder. Often caused by swimming or extensive overhead work.

Lateral Collateral Ligament: The ligament on the outside of the knee that connects the femur with the fibula.

Lower extremity compartment syndrome: can be caused by acute trauma or exercise, resulting in an increased pressure to one of the compartments in lower leg. Can occasionally be a medical emergency.

Medial Collateral Ligament: the large ligament on the inside of the knee that connects the femur to the tibia.

Medial Tibial Stress Syndrome: commonly called shin splints, an overuse injury of the shin area, primarily inside the tibia.

Meniscectomy: usually refers to the surgical removal of the torn part of the meniscus.

Meniscus: the cartilaginous disc found in the knee. There is a medial and lateral meniscus. Torn menisci are usually removed arthroscopically. Loss of the meniscus is often a precursor to osteoarthritis.

Myositis Ossificans: when bone (calcified) tissue forms inside muscle usually as a result of trauma. The thigh and upper arm are the most common sites.

Osgood Schlatter's Disease (OSD): inflammation of the patella tendon primarily at the top and front of the tibia. OSD is more common during growth in children.

Osteoarthritis: the most common form of arthritis. Occurs when the articular cartilage on the ends of bones is worn by excessive use or injury.

Osteoporosis: reduction in the density of bone leading to a host of problems.

Overtraining Syndrome: a condition brought about by long-term intense training coupled with reduced rest. The result is reduced performance. Athletes with overtraining syndrome may take months to recover.

Patella: the small bone in front of the knee that connects the quadricep muscles to the tibia via the patella tendon.

Periodization: a planned training program using a manipulation of intensity and volume to bring about peak performance. Planned rest is part of periodization.

Periosteum: the outer layer of bone.

Physiatrist: a medical doctor who practices physical medicine and rehabilitation largely through physical therapy and medication.

Plantar Fasciitis: inflammation of the plantar fascia on the bottom of the foot. The most common cause of heel pain.

Plyometrics: a training program designed to enhance the stretch-shortening cycle (SSC) of the muscle/tendon contraction. Box jumping (jumping off one box onto another) is a common form of plyometrics.

Posterior Cruciate Ligament: the small ligament in the middle of the knee that connects the back of the tibia with the front of the femur. Works with the ACL to provide anterior/posterior stability.

Rotator Cuff: the four small muscles that originate off the scapula and surround the head of the humerus providing stabilization and rotation.

Secondary Impact Syndrome: a serious condition in which an individual has a second concussion before the symptoms of the first concussion are gone.

Separated Shoulder: a sprain or rupture of the acromioclavicular ligament, the ligament that connects the scapula to the clavicle.

Sever's Disease: an injury to the growth plate on the back of the calcaneus (heel) where the Achilles tendon attaches. Like Osgood Schlatter's disease, this injury often occurs during growth.

Sprain: an injury to the ligaments surrounding a joint.

Subluxation: a temporary dislocation of a joint in which the dislocation is reduced without outside manipulation.

Tendinosis: an overuse injury to a tendon in which there is disruption in the pathology of the tendon not normally caused by inflammation.

Tendonitis: inflammation of a tendon such as that occurring with tennis elbow or golfer's elbow.

Tibia: the large shin bone.

Tuberosity: a secondary growth on a bone to accommodate the attachment of tendons or ligaments, sometimes called a secondary epiphysis.

Ulnar Collateral Ligament: the ligament on the inside of the elbow that is damaged with frequent high-speed throwing. This is the ligament that is replaced with Tommy John surgery.

Unhappy Triad: a combination of a torn medial collateral ligament, medial meniscus, and ACL.

VO_{2max}: the maximum amount of oxygen one can consume in a minute. This is commonly used as the default value for aerobic power.

Directory of Resources

BOOKS

Achar, S., & Taylor K. *The 5-Minute Sports Medicine Consult*, 3rd ed. Philadelphia: Wolters Kluwer, 2019.

Boyle, M. *Advances in Functional Training*. Apto, CA: On Target Publications, 2010.

Boyle, M. *New Functional Training for Sport*, 2nd ed. Champaign, IL: Human Kinetics, 2016.

Buschbacher R., Prahlow, N., & Shashank, J. *Sports Medicine and Rehabilitation: A Sport-Specific Approach*. Philadelphia: Lippincott, 2009.

Delavier, F. *Strength Training Anatomy*, 3d ed. Champaign, IL: Human Kinetics, 2010.

Haff, F., & Triplett, N., eds. *Essentials of Strength Training and Conditioning*, 4th ed. Champaign, IL: Human Kinetics, 2016.

Joyce, D., & Lewindon, D., eds. *Sports Injury Prevention and Rehabilitation*. New York: Routledge, 2016.

McGill, S. *Low Back Disorders*. Champaign, IL: Human Kinetics, 2007.

McGill, S. *Ultimate Back Fitness and Performance*, 6th ed. BackFitPro.com, 2017.

WEBSITES

American College of Sports Medicine—the primary organization for sports medicine research in the United States.
   https://www.acsm.org/

Bicycle Helmet Safety Institute—provides a rating system for helmets.
   https://helmets.org/

FIFA warm-up—a program to warm up and reduce injury.
   https://www.kort.com/uploadedFiles/KORT/Content/Services/Sports
   _Medicine/Concussion_Management/FIFA-the-11-Booklet.pdf

Hip Mobility Exercises—video of exercises designed to improve hip mobility.
   https://drjohnrusin.com/10-exercises-to-instantly-improve-hip
   -mobility/

McGill's Big 3 Core Stability Exercises—a video of McGill's exercises to increase the stability of the trunk.
   https://www.youtube.com/watch?v=S8VFbkSjCsQ

National Athletic Trainer's Association—the organization of accredited athletic trainers in the United States.
   https://www.nata.org/

National Strength and Conditioning Association—an organization that presents applied exercise science research and accreditation for strength and conditioning specialists.
   https://www.nsca.com/

National Weather Service Heat Index.
   https://www.weather.gov/safety/heat-index

PEP Program—a description of knee stability program in Santa Monica, CA.
   https://www.aclstudygroup.com/pdf/pep-program.pdf

Rating Site for Hospitals—a site that rates hospitals that might help when a surgery is necessary.
   https://www.medicare.gov/hospitalcompare/search.html?#

Rating Site for Surgeons—this rating system of surgeons across the country might help when selecting a surgeon.
https://www.checkbook.org/surgeonratings/default.cfm

Rotator Cuff Exercises—a set of exercises one can use to stretch and strengthen the four muscles that compose the rotator cuff.
https://www.healthline.com/health/rotator-cuff-injury-stretches

Shoulder Mobility Routine—an excellent video of exercises one can utilize to improve shoulder flexibility.
https://www.youtube.com/watch?v=3g95hw1QMmY

Sportsmetrics Cincinnati, OH—the website for the organization that does a considerable amount of research on anterior cruciate ligament injury prevention.
https://sportsmetrics.org/

Thrower's Ten—description and analysis of a set of 10 exercises anyone can use who tends to throw or hit overhand.
https://www.muhlenberg.edu/media/contentassets/pdf/athletics/athletictraining/throwers10.pdf

Index

About the Author

James H. Johnson, PhD, is professor emeritus of Smith College in Northampton, Massachusetts. He started his professional career at Louisiana State University, where he received a PhD and worked as an athletic trainer for football, basketball, and track and field athletes. After stints as a teacher at the University of South Alabama and Washington University in St. Louis, he settled at Smith College. He has worked as a professor of exercise and sport for 52 years, published numerous articles in peer-review journals, and spoken widely on injury prevention. At Smith he was instrumental in creating the award-winning graduate program in coaching education.